The Profession
of
Dietetics

FIFTH EDITION

A TEAM APPROACH

June R. Payne-Palacio, PhD, RD
Professor Emeritus
Pepperdine University

Deborah D. Canter, PhD, RD, LD
Professor
Department of Hospitality Management and Dietetics
Kansas State University

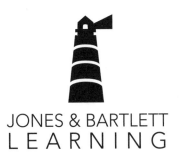

JONES & BARTLETT
LEARNING

World Headquarters
Jones & Bartlett Learning
5 Wall Street
Burlington, MA 01803
978-443-5000
info@jblearning.com
www.jblearning.com

Jones & Bartlett Learning books and products are available through most bookstores and online booksellers. To contact Jones & Bartlett Learning directly, call 800-832-0034, fax 978-443-8000, or visit our website, www.jblearning.com.

Production Credits

Publisher: William Brottmiller
Editorial Assistant: Agnes Burt
Production Editor: Joanna Lundeen
Senior Marketing Manager: Andrea DeFronzo
VP, Manufacturing and Inventory Control:
  Therese Connell
Composition: Lapiz, Inc.
Cover Designer: Michael O'Donnell
Rights & Photo Research Assistant: Joseph Veiga

Cover Images: (nutrition counseling a patient) © Creatas/
  Thinkstock; (MyPlate overlay) Courtesy of USDA;
  (dietitian with children) © Courtesy of Peggy Greb/USDA;
  (dietitian and patient) Photo by Scott Bauer/USDA;
  (news interview) © Bruce C. Murray/ShutterStock, Inc.;
  (background) © Veronika Vasilyuk/ShutterStock, Inc.
Title Page Image: © Veronika Vasilyuk/ShutterStock, Inc.
Printing and Binding: Edwards Brothers Malloy
Cover Printing: Edwards Brothers Malloy

To order this product, use ISBN: 978-1-284-02608-5

Library of Congress Cataloging-in-Publication Data
Payne-Palacio, June.
  The profession of dietetics : a team approach / by June Payne-Palacio and Deborah Canter.—5th ed.
    p. ; cm.
  Includes bibliographical references and index.
  ISBN 978-1-4496-7838-8 -- ISBN 1-4496-7838-6
  I. Canter, Deborah D.   II. Title.
  [DNLM: 1. Dietetics—education.   2. Dietetics—methods.   3. Patient Care Team.   WB 400]
  613.2023—dc23

                                    2012046659

6048

Printed in the United States of America
17 16 15 14   10 9 8 7 6 5 4 3

BRIEF CONTENTS

CONTENTS

CHAPTER 10   Crossing the Bridge: From Student to Professional   201

APPENDIX   Commonly Used Acronyms in the Dietetics Profession   217

Index   221

The Profession of Dietetics: A Team Approach is written for students interested in finding out more about the profession of dietetics. Understanding who dietetics professionals are, what dietetics professionals do, and how to become a certified dietary manager; a dietetic technician, registered; or a registered dietitian is a complex task. Few other professions offer so many educational routes for entry or so many ways to practice one's trade. While this diversity is a strength, it often confuses those who wish to enter the profession, as well as prospective customers who are trying to understand who dietetics professionals are or why they should consult one.

It is the goal of this book to present a clear and up-to-date picture of the profession of dietetics and to try to answer some basic questions:

- What is a profession and how does dietetics qualify as a profession?
- How has the history of the profession shaped dietetics practice today?
- Who are members of the dietetics team and how do they work together?
- What is the Academy of Nutrition and Dietetics (formerly the American Dietetic Association) and why should one become a member?
- What is credentialing of dietetics professionals and why is it important?
- What kinds of positions do dietetics professionals fill?
- Why are communication and teamwork so important in the dietetics profession?
- How can a person develop effective communication skills and become a good team player?
- What are some ways to successfully make the transition from student to professional?
- What does the future hold for dietetics practice?

Features throughout the text are designed to help students connect with the material presented. Suggested Activities at the end of each chapter allow students to explore topics further and offer opportunities for thought-provoking research outside the classroom. Selected websites direct students to view related content online and to peruse a variety of Web pages pertaining to the field of dietetics. The ever-popular Profile of a Professional feature includes real interviews with individuals who work in various positions as dietetics professionals.

Each professional who is profiled offers advice and words of wisdom for students entering the field.

This edition also features a Navigate Companion Website, go.jblearning .com/ProfessionOfDietetics5e, where readers can access relevant and up-to-date supplementary information. Student resources include Web Links and an Interactive Glossary. Instructor resources include PowerPoint Presentations, Instructor's Manual, and a Test Bank.

The profession of dietetics is dynamic, exciting, and in need of enthusiastic, energetic, and visionary men and women who wish to join the team. It is our hope that this book enlightens, informs, and inspires those who read it. If this occurs, then our dream for this book will have been achieved.

ACKNOWLEDGMENTS

We owe a debt of gratitude to Karen Lechowich at the Academy of Nutrition and Dietetics who, because of her love of this profession and its history, went "above and beyond the call of duty" in her efforts to help us with this project. We would also like to express special thanks to our editorial and production staff at Jones & Bartlett Learning for their patience while working with us and for their support and encouragement for the completion of this revision; William Brottmiller, Agnes Burt, and Joanna Lundeen pushed and prodded us at the right times, always with tact and diplomacy, to make sure this book was published on time. Their guidance and wise suggestions made this a better book.

We wish to acknowledge the special people in our lives who helped us through the production of this edition. Appreciation is expressed to Deb's "adopted family," Rebecca and Jeff Daniels and children Hope, Ian, Grace, Nigel, and Gavin in Kansas City, and friends Sharon and Medo Morcos in Manhattan, who share so much love and support. Special love and appreciation is also expressed to June's husband, Cliff Duboff, for his emotional support and untiring help. And, finally, we thank the dietetics students at Pepperdine University, Kansas State University, and across the country who daily confirm our belief in the secure future of the profession of dietetics.

The Past

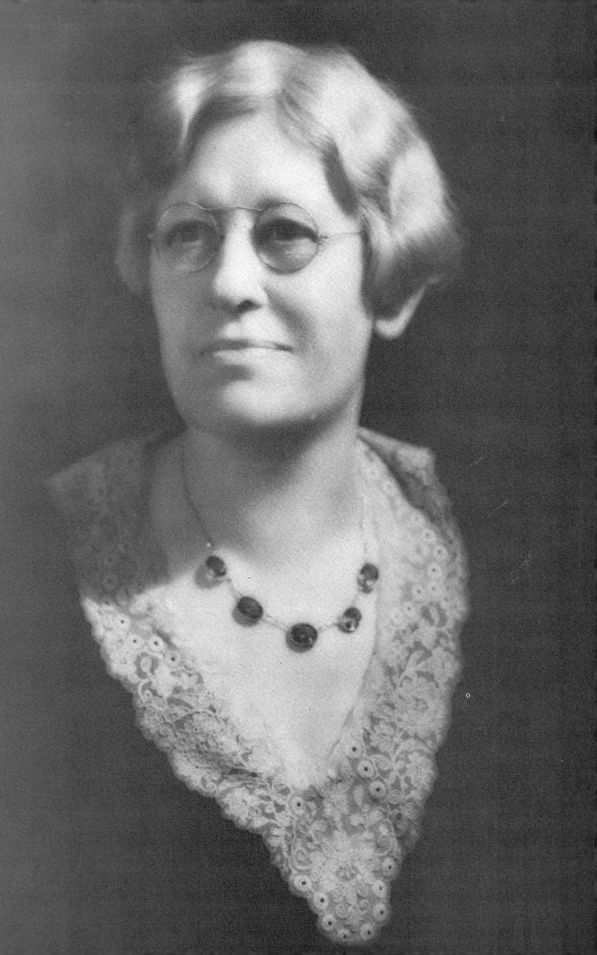

The Profession Is Born

The Very Beginning

Why begin with the history of the dietetics profession? History provides people with an opportunity to learn from past mistakes and can also show which of the seeds that were sown blossomed into successes and why. As stated on Radford University's Department of History website:

> *The study of history provides a window into the past that provides understanding of the present day, and how individuals, nations, and the global community might develop in the future. Historical study instructs how societies came to be and examines cultural, political, social, and economic influences across time and space.*[1]

The profession of dietetics, although relatively young, has an interesting, rich, and diverse past that stems from the much older history of food and health. Some very old sayings advise "An ounce of prevention is worth a pound of cure" and "An apple a day keeps the doctor away." The role of food in preventing, curing, treating, or causing illness has been recognized since the beginning of recorded human history. "If a man has pain inside, food and drink coming back to his mouth . . . let him refrain from eating onions for three days" is the first known written dietary recommendation, carved on Babylonian stone tablets around 2500 B.C.[2] The typical daily regimen during this time consisted of barley paste or bread, onions, a few beans, and beer.

The Book of Judges in the Old Testament contains a prenatal dietary prescription that has withstood the test of time: "Therefore beware, and drink no wine or strong drink, and eat nothing unclean, for lo, you shall conceive and bear a son."[3] The Book of Daniel contains what is probably the first controlled dietary experiment. Daniel and the other young men from Judah asked their guards to allow them to maintain their ancestral traditions and eat pulses (legumes) and bread and drink water rather than the king's rich food and wine allowance for 10 days. At the end of the 10 days, they were healthier and better nourished than all the young men who had lived on the food assigned to them by the king.[4]

Scurvy, which is caused by a vitamin C deficiency, was described as early as 1500 B.C. in the Ebers Papyrus, and other descriptions appear in ancient Greek and Roman writings.[5] The word *diet* is from the Greek *diatta*, which means "manner of living."[6] It appears in many early writings, including those of Hippocrates and Galen.[7] The oldest known cookbook, Apicius's *De Re Culinaria* (approximately 100 B.C.), contains many dietary principles that are still sound today.[8] One entire book of the 10 books contained in the cookbook attributed to Apicius is devoted to pulses, or legumes, which are mentioned in the Old Testament. In ancient China, food therapy was practiced as a special branch of medicine.[9] Chinese observations about diabetes date to the third century, and descriptions of night blindness and its correct dietary cure date to the seventh century.[10,11]

The Middle Ages

During the Song Dynasty (960–1279) in China, Ben Cao Tu Jing, in the *Atlas of Materia Medica* (1061), described a "clinical trial" to determine the efficacy of ginseng. He suggested, "In order to evaluate the efficacy of ginseng, find two people and let one eat ginseng and run, and the other run without ginseng. The one that did not eat ginseng will develop shortness of breath sooner."[12]

William the Conqueror was probably one of the first famous names in history to go on a weight-loss diet. In 1087, he tried to lose weight by going on a liquid diet, taking to his bed and consuming nothing but alcohol!

Hospital records from St. Bartholomew's Hospital (**Figure 1–1**), which was founded in Britain in 1123, provide the first written evidence of a typical hospital menu. Bread and beer formed the basis of the diet.[13] This obviously inadequate and unpalatable diet led to a prevalence of **scurvy** (a condition characterized by weakness, joint pain, skin lesions and bruising, bleeding gums, and loosening of teeth) among patients. Other conditions in early British hospitals were also poor. Sanitation was nonexistent, overcrowding was common, buildings were unsafe, and stern disciplinary measures were used on noncompliant patients.

With the publication of *De re Medicina* in 1478 in Florence, Italy, diet became an important part of medical practice. In this publication, medicine was divided into three branches: diseases treated manually, diseases treated by medicine, and diseases treated by diet. In 1480, the first printed cookbook appeared, containing reference to quality and varieties of meat, fish, fruits, and vegetables; information on how they nourish the body; and directions on how they should be prepared.[14]

Weight-loss books appeared in the late 1600s to early 1700s. A Scotsman, Dr. George Cheyne, wrote two popular books, *An Essay of Health and Long Life* and *The English Malady*, in which he described a milk diet, which he claimed, kept him "lank, fleet and nimble."[15]

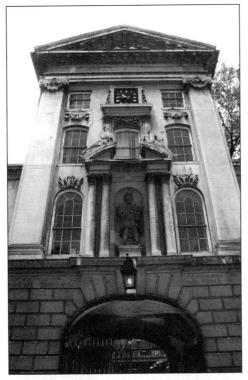

FIGURE 1–1 St. Bartholomew's Hospital, London.
Courtesy of Barts and the London NHS Trust

Progress (?) in the Eighteenth and Nineteenth Centuries

The first hospitals in the United States were in Philadelphia—Philadelphia General Hospital was built in 1731 and Pennsylvania Hospital (**Figure 1–2**) was built in 1751.[13] In these hospitals, little thought was given to food, and conditions were very poor. Mush and molasses were the usual fare, with a pint of beer included for supper.[16] After the War of 1812; fruit was added to the menu as a garnish.

Until the eighteenth century, beliefs and writings about diet were based on insufficient scientific evidence. But with advances in chemistry and physics came the foundation necessary to establish dietetics as a profession. The work of Antoine-Laurent de Lavoisier (1743–1794) on digestion is generally regarded as the first modern, scientific research on nutrition (**Figure 1–3**). The son of a wealthy Parisian lawyer, Lavoisier was trained as a lawyer. Chemistry was his hobby.[17]

Nutritional epidemiology, the study of the relationship of diet to human disease, is often dated to 1747, the same year as the earliest known clinical trial was conducted by Dr. James Lind (**Figure 1–4**). Lind was the ship doctor on the HMS *Salisbury* when it set sail from England to the Plymouth Colony. During this time, scurvy and typhoid were often responsible for the deaths of more than half of the crewmembers of sailing ships. A British report

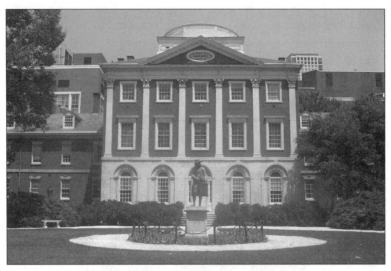

Figure 1–2 Pennsylvania Hospital, one of the first hospitals in the United States.
Copyright © 2006 by Sarah B. Hecht

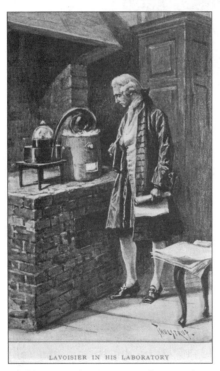

LAVOISIER IN HIS LABORATORY

Figure 1–3 Antoine Lavoisier is shown with the chemistry apparatus he used to study digestion.
Courtesy of the National Library of Medicine

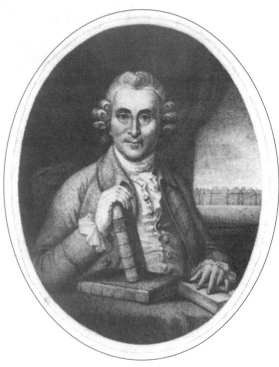

Figure 1–4 A portrait of James Lind holding his book *Lind on Scurvy.*
Courtesy of the Royal College of Physicians of Edinburgh

in 1600 indicated that in the previous 20 years more than 10,000 mariners had died from scurvy alone. On board the *Salisbury*, Lind took 12 men ill with scurvy and divided them into six groups of two each. All ate the same food for breakfast, lunch, and dinner, but each group received a different supplement each day:

1. Quart of apple juice
2. Twenty-five drops of elixir vitriol (sulfuric acid and aromatics)
3. Two spoonfuls of vinegar three times a day
4. Concoction of herbs and spices
5. Half-pint of seawater daily
6. Two oranges and one lemon

The two men who ate the oranges and lemons recovered almost immediately. Both were fit enough to return to work in 6 days, and one became the nurse to the others. The two who drank the apple juice improved, but were not well enough to work. None of the others showed any improvement. Lind concluded that citrus fruit contained something that counteracted the ravages of scurvy; he gave all the men oranges and lemons and they were cured. This discovery was followed by the development of a method for the concentration and preservation of citrus fruit juices for use at sea. In 1795, the British Royal Navy provided a daily ration of lemon or lime juice as an **antiscorbutic** (protects against scurvy). Because at the time both lemons and limes were called limes, Americans and Australians began to call English ships and sailors "lime-juicers," and later "limeys." Much later, a deficiency of vitamin C, ascorbic acid, was determined to be the cause of scurvy.[5]

Still, progress was slow. A patient in an English hospital in the eighteenth century would receive the only menu served each day:

- Four to five ounces of meat (usually already boiled for the broth)
- Three-quarters to 1 pound of bread
- Two to three pints of beer
- Pottage or pudding

Fruits and vegetables were missing from this daily allowance—they were suspected by some as being harmful and by others as having medicinal, rather than nutritive, value. Small amounts of cheese, butter, roots, and greens were sometimes included in the daily fare. Family and friends could bring food to supplement the meager hospital offerings or patients could buy food from the food sellers who came through the wards.

The most expensive item on the menu was beer. Doctors at the time believed that alcohol was necessary to treat illness. Because water often was contaminated, beer was used extensively. When cost-cutting measures were instituted, the beer allowance was reduced or completely eliminated.

Patients who were unable to eat the full diet or who complained about the food were disciplined. Punishments included cutting the food allowance in half, omitting some meals entirely, or restricting patients to toast and water for a week.[18]

Meanwhile, famous individuals continued to go on diets, and other individuals became famous because of the diets they promoted. In 1811 the romantic poet Lord Byron reduced his weight from 194 to 130 pounds by drenching his food in vinegar. In the 1830s in the United States, the Reverend Sylvester Graham, nicknamed "Dr. Sawdust," railed against the sin of gluttony, which he said led to lust, indigestion, and the rearing of unhealthy children. His recommended spartan diet included coarse, yeast-free, brown bread (including his famous Graham cracker), vegetables, and water.[15]

Little improvement in hospital conditions occurred until the humanitarian movement of the late nineteenth century. Great progress was made between 1850 and 1920.

Florence Nightingale (1820–1910) (**Figure 1–5**), a superintendent of nurses in British military hospitals in Turkey during the Crimean War (1854–1856), established foodservice for the troops. With the help of a French chef, Alexis Soyer, she reduced the death rate of injured soldiers by improving diet and sanitary conditions. Later, in her writings and nursing practice, Nightingale continued to demonstrate her belief in the importance of nutrition and foodservice management by emphasizing the selection and service of food and the art and science of feeding the sick.[19]

At around the same time, the low-carbohydrate, high-protein diet was first introduced. London undertaker William Banting lost 50 pounds on a high-protein regimen consisting of lean meat, dry toast, soft-boiled eggs, and vegetables. His 1864 book, *Letter on Corpulence*, became a bestseller, and by 1880 "Banting" had become the foremost American weight-loss strategy. Yet another proponent of high-protein diets, Dr. James Salisbury, recommended minced meat patties (what we know as Salisbury steaks) and hot water for improving health and aiding weight loss.[15]

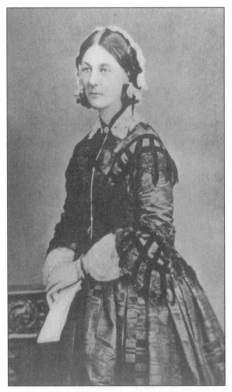

FIGURE 1–5 A portrait of Florence Nightingale.
Courtesy of Library of Congress, Prints & Photographs Division [reproduction number cph.3a09175]

The Iowa Agriculture School in Ames in 1872 was probably the first college to offer courses in cookery. A yearly course in "household chemistry," which included cookery, was started in 1877 at the Kansas State Agricultural College in Manhattan.[20] Other colleges and universities soon followed their lead.

In 1876 Dr. John Harvey Kellogg became the staff physician of the Battle Creek Sanitarium in Michigan. Kellogg invented granola and toasted flakes, for which his name is well known. At the time, he was known as a diet guru who crusaded for vegetarianism, pure foods, slow chewing, calorie counting, colon cleansing, and individualized diets.[15]

The first American dietitian is considered to be Sarah Tyson Rorer (1849–1937) (**Figure 1–6**). Her training consisted of some medical school lectures and a 3-month cooking course. In 1878 Rorer opened the Philadelphia Cooking School where students learned about food values, protein, and carbohydrates, but nothing about calories and vitamins. Students took 10 classes in chemistry, several in physiology and hygiene, and 10 on cooking for the sick. Twelve students graduated each year for 33 years, and they secured positions planning meals and supervising production in hospital kitchens.[21]

In 1877, the American Medical Association formed a Committee on Dietetics and asked Rorer to edit a new publication entitled *The Dietetic Gazette*.[22] Later, she published *Household News* on her own, in which she wrote articles on topics such as feeding the sick and designing a kitchen and answered readers' diet-related questions.[23] In her lifetime, she authored more than 50 books and booklets and wrote articles for such magazines as *Ladies' Home Journal*, *Table Talk*, and *Good Housekeeping*.[24] Rorer also established the first diet kitchen and dietary counseling service, at the request of three well-known physicians.

Meanwhile the popular diets continued to evolve. Milk diets, earlier prescribed for indigestion and weight gain, now became popular for weight loss. Dr. Edward Hooker Dewey recommended skipping breakfast and a moderate

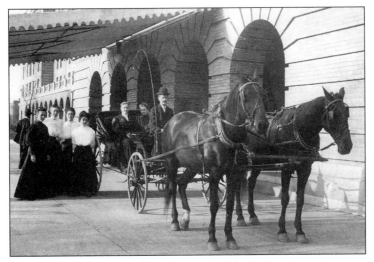

FIGURE 1–6 Sarah Tyson Rorer, first American dietitian (left) and Lenna Frances Cooper (right) in a carriage at the Battle Creek Sanitarium.
Courtesy of the Academy of Nutrition and Dietetics

fast as a weight-loss strategy. Other doctors of the time touted substituting carbohydrates with protein and limiting consumption of alcohol.[15]

Previously thought to be an infectious disease, beriberi received attention from several researchers around the world. In 1884, Kanehiro Takaki linked Japanese sailors' diet of polished rice to the disease **beriberi** (a condition characterized by weakness in the legs, hands, and arms and, later, weakening of the cardiac muscles, leading to heart failure). By adding milk and vegetables to the sailors' diet, he eliminated the disease.[25] In 1889, Christiaan Eijkman in the Dutch East Indies took the research one step further by proposing a nutritional hypothesis for the cause of beriberi. His experimentation with chickens led to the conclusion that unpolished rice contained an "anti-beriberi factor."[26] As with vitamin C, the identification of vitamin B_1 as the deficient nutrient came much later.

In 1896, the U.S. Department of Agriculture (USDA) published *Bulletin 28*, which featured the first food composition tables.[27] The *Bulletin* was an indispensable resource for dietetic practitioners for many years.

In 1898, when businessman Horace Fletcher was denied life insurance because of his weight, he lost 40 pounds by chewing every mouthful of food to liquefy it before swallowing. The slow-chewing movement (Fletcherism) took off, supported by diet guru Kellogg, whose patients were instructed to chew every mouthful of food 32 times before swallowing. This became known as "Fletcherizing."[15]

At the Lake Placid Conference on Home Economics in 1899, the term *dietitian* was first defined. The conference attendees determined that the title **dietitian** should be "applied to persons who specialize in the knowledge of food and can meet the demands of the medical profession for diet therapy."[28]

The Young Profession in the Twentieth Century

Florence Corbett established the first internship for dietitians in 1903 at the New York Department of Charities. Applicants for the 3-month course had to be older than 25 years of age, have 1 year of teaching experience, and be a domestic science graduate.[7]

In 1907, an English doctor, William Fletcher, conducted an experiment on inmates of a lunatic asylum in Kuala Lumpur, Malaysia, which provided definitive proof that certain types of rice were either the direct or indirect cause of beriberi. His experiment was rigorous and mimicked several features of a modern randomized trial.[26]

Working at the famed Lister Institute in London in 1912, Casimir Funk (1884–1967), a Polish-born biochemist, took Fletcher's thinking to the next level. He isolated the active substances in the husks of unpolished rice that were preventing beriberi and named them *amines*, because he believed they were derived from ammonia. Because these substances appeared essential for life, he added the prefix *vita*. Later, he postulated the existence of four such substances (B_1, B_2, C, and D), which he stated were necessary for normal health and for the prevention of deficiency diseases. Discovery and synthesis of all of the individual vitamins would come much later, but this initial discovery was a milestone in nutritional history.[29]

In 1910, dietitians were practicing in poorly defined roles with a diversity of titles. Few people could define the role of the *dietist, dietician, dietitian,* or *nutrition worker,* as dietitians were variously called. The title *nutritionist* appeared in the early 1920s, and the spelling of *dietitian* was agreed upon in 1930.[30]

Fighting faddism and quackery was an issue in 1910, just as it is today. Fletcherizing was just one example of a harmless but ineffective popular notion of that day. Calorie counting, high-protein or low-protein diets, and natural foods were other popular fads. Food scales, developed for diabetics, became central to diet plans.

Nutritional research received an unexpected boost in importance with the outbreak of World War I. The examination of 2.5 million military draftees in Great Britain in 1917 found 41% to be in poor health and unfit for duty, most commonly because of nutritional status.[31] In the United States, the American Red Cross enrolled dietitians for military duty. The initial qualifications were 2 years of college study majoring in home economics and 4 months of practical experience in hospital dietetics. The National Committee on Dietitian Service of the American Red Cross established these qualifications. The first military dietitian to serve overseas was deployed in May 1917. In World War I, 356 dietitians served in the armed services.[32] Mary Pascoe Huddleson, a dietitian with Base Hospitals No. 8, No. 117, and No. 214, was among them. The nutritional expertise of these brave dietitians provided leadership for both the nourishment of hospitalized soldiers and the general public at home. Conservation of food was encouraged, and dietitians advised the government on efficient methods of food production, distribution, and preparation.

When the American Home Economic Association decided not to hold its annual meeting in 1917 because of the war, two dietitians, Lenna Frances Cooper (previously shown in **Figure 1–6**) and Lulu G. Graves (**Figure 1–7**),

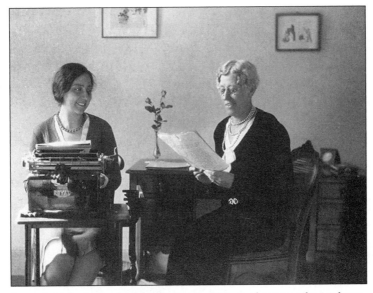

FIGURE 1–7 Lulu Graves, first president of the ADA, now known as the Academy of Nutrition and Dietetics, in her office with her assistant.
Courtesy of the Academy of Nutrition and Dietetics

organized a special meeting of hospital dietitians to discuss emergency war needs. Out of the meeting of 98 people, the American Dietetic Association (ADA) was formed (**Figure 1–8**). This association, with 39 charter members and dues of $1 per year, was formed to address the interests of dietitians. Its first president was Lulu Graves, who was head of the department at Lakeside Hospital in Cleveland (**Figure 1–9**). The first meeting of the ADA (now known as the Academy of Nutrition and Dietetics) was held in the basement at Lakeside Hospital. Graves served as president for the first 3 years. Lenna Frances Cooper served as the first vice president.[7]

In 1918, *Diet and Health with a Key to the Calories*, written by the best-known and best-loved woman physician in America—Dr. Lulu Hunt Peters—was a bestseller. The diet began with a fast and then transitioned

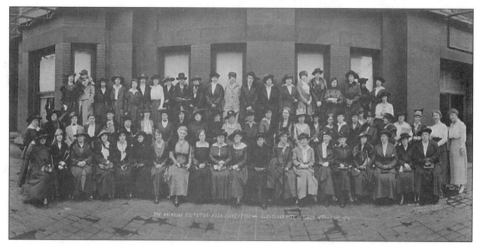

FIGURE 1–8 Attendees at the 1917 conference where the ADA, now known as the Academy of Nutrition and Dietetics, was founded.
Courtesy of the Academy of Nutrition and Dietetics

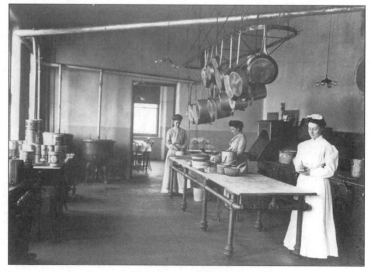

FIGURE 1–9 Lakeside Hospital kitchen, 1905. The first meeting of the American Dietetic Association was held in the basement of this hospital in 1917.
Courtesy of the Academy of Nutrition and Dietetics

to Fletcherism and calorie counting, with a 1,200-calorie-a-day regimen prescribed for life.[15]

Dieto-therapy as practiced in the early 1900s consisted of many special diets, such as the Sippy Diet for ulcers, which consisted of cream and poached eggs. Diabetic diets varied widely, even after the discovery of insulin in 1921. Doctors prescribed very low-calorie diets of 600 to 750 calories a day for severely obese patients beginning in 1928. Ten years later, the regimen was reduced to 400 calories a day.

The 1920s saw a dizzying array of food-limiting regimens. The 18-day Hollywood diet allowed 585 calories a day, limited mostly to grapefruit, oranges, eggs, and Melba toast. The lamb chop and the pineapple diets were also popular. The first food-combining diet was introduced, in which dieters were admonished not to combine starches, fruits, and proteins in the same meal.[15]

On a more scientific level, the successful treatment of pernicious anemia with a special diet was reported in the *Journal of the American Medical Association*.[33] The passage of the federal Maternity and Infancy Act in the 1920s allowed state health departments to employ nutritionists.[30] The passage of Title V of the Social Security Act in 1935 provided major impetus for the employment of nutrition consultants in state and local health departments by making federal funds available for this purpose.[30,34]

In 1922, the Medical Department Professional Service Schools at Walter Reed General Hospital was established, becoming the first Army training program for dietitians. The program met ADA requirements and was the only training course provided for dietitians by the Army from 1922 to 1942 (**Figure 1–10**). World War II contributed to the public recognition of the role of dietitians. Nearly 2,000 dietitians were commissioned in the armed services, and many others educated the public at home. The practice of dietetics

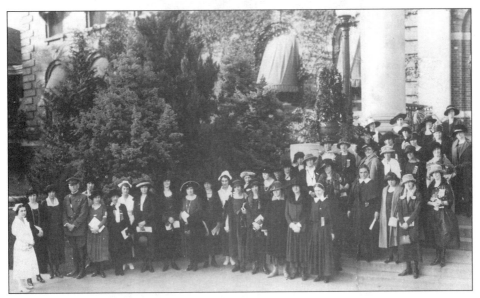

FIGURE 1–10 Dietitians at Walter Reed General Hospital in 1922.
Courtesy of the Academy of Nutrition and Dietetics

broadened to include institutions such as restaurants, airlines, and industrial plants. After the war, dietitians were granted full military status, and their position in the healthcare setting was strengthened with the emphasis on allied health professions and the healthcare team concept.[7]

Passage of the National School Lunch Act in 1946 expanded dietetics to include the establishment of school lunch programs, including the training of personnel in foodservice and nutrition education. The Hill-Burton Hospital Facilities Survey and Construction Act (1946) and the Medicare and Medicaid legislation of the 1960s created demand for the services of consultant dietitians in healthcare facilities such as nursing homes.[34]

In 1948, Take Off Pounds Sensibly (TOPS) became the first national group dieting organization. The TOPS program focused on calories, scales, food diaries, and mutual support. Still going strong, TOPS has added physical activity and the use of exchange lists to its weight-loss program.[15]

Dietitians were actively recruited for service during the Korean War (**Figure 1–11**). At this time, the role of the military dietitian started to expand to include not only therapeutic dietetics, but also the supervision and operation of the entire hospital foodservice.[32]

Overeaters Anonymous was founded in 1960 and Weight Watchers in 1961. During this same time, Mead Johnson introduced a diet formula, Metrecal, whose success spawned many imitators. The 1960s saw a number

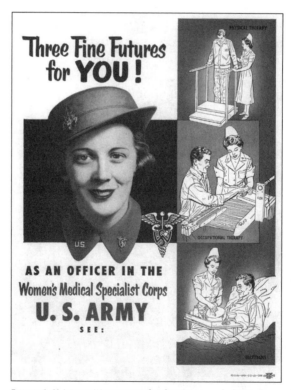

FIGURE 1–11 A recruiting poster for dietitians and physical and occupational therapists during the Korean War.
Women's Medical Specialist Corps recruiting poster. U.S. War Poster Collection (MSS044), Betty H. Carter Women Veterans Historical Project, University of North Carolina at Greensboro, NC, USA

of diet book bestsellers. Touting the low-carbohydrate, high-protein diets were *Calories Don't Count* and *The Doctor's Quick Weight Loss Diet*. In the alcohol-friendly, low-carbohydrate category were *The Drinking Man's Diet* and *Martinis and Whipped Cream*.[15]

The civil rights movement of the 1960s brought the issues of poverty and hunger into the political spotlight. The government instituted its war on poverty, and Senator Hubert Humphrey worked with the Senate Select Committee on Nutrition and Human Needs.[35] As a result of these and other efforts, USDA food assistance programs to low-income families were established or expanded in the 1970s. Important among these were the Food Stamp Program and school lunch and breakfast programs; child care and summer foodservice for children; supplemental feeding programs for women, infants, and children (WIC); and nutrition for the elderly.[36]

During the Vietnam conflict, 26 Army dietitians were assigned to all four combat tactical zones. They formulated meals for hospital patients on modified diets, planned the basic troop-issue menus for all Army personnel in the country, and implemented the menus for all personnel in medical treatment facilities. These tasks were complicated by the fact that in 1966 there were 385,000 troops in Vietnam and refrigeration was minimal. Air Force dietitians developed a system to order, prepare, and serve therapeutic in-flight meals for patients who were being evacuated from combat zones.[37]

Food assistance programs have developed more rapidly and with more support than nutrition education programs. In 1968, the Cooperative Extension Service of the USDA began the Expanded Food and Nutrition Education Program (EFNEP), which provides nutrition and food education for low-income families. In 1975, 3 years after the start of the WIC program, an education component was legislated. And, in 1977, nutrition education was incorporated into the Food Stamp Program. The Food and Agriculture Act of 1977 included the Nutrition Education and Training Program (NETP or NET), the first federal nutrition program for children.[36] The Academy of Nutrition and Dietetics and others expressed the need for making nutrition education a primary component of all food assistance programs.[38]

As the general public continued to seek ways to lose weight quickly and easily, a steady stream of diet books rolled off the presses (**Table 1–1**). Most were slight variations on old themes.

Entering the Twenty-First Century

In 2003, *The South Beach Diet* hit the bookstores. It is a moderate diet falling midway between the low-fat, high-carbohydrate recommendations of trained dietitians and the low-carbohydrate, high-protein Atkins diet.

Today, dietetics is an honored profession with members striving to achieve the highest professional standards of integrity, service, competence, and vision. Two leaders of the profession wrote recently:

> *Our profession today is marked by achievement and change . . .*
> *[We] have come a long way in a relatively short period of time. We*
> *have become valued professional members of health-care teams and*

TABLE 1–1

Timeline of Late Twentieth-Century Diets

1970s   Astronauts' diet—liquid meals.

1972   *Dr. Atkins' Diet Revolution*—lots of meat. Carbohydrates are banned.

1976   *The Last Chance Diet*—fasting and liquid drinks made from animal tendons and hides. Fifty-eight deaths were attributed to these and similar liquid formulas that lack essential nutrients.

1978   *Scarsdale Diet*—high protein, 700 calories per day.

1979   *Pritikin Program for Diet and Exercise*—very low-fat regimen.

1981   *The Beverly Hills Diet*—food-combining diet with lots of fruit.

1983   Jenny Craig is founded.

1992   *Dr. Atkins' New Diet Revolution.*

1993   *Eat More, Weigh Less*—low-fat, vegetarian diet.

1995   *The Zone*—low-carbohydrate, high-protein diet soon joined by *Sugar Busters, Protein Power,* and *The Carbohydrate Addicts' Diet.*

1996   *The New Beverly Hills Diet* (see 1981).

1998   *Lose Weight with Apple Vinegar*—Lord Byron's strategy resurfaces!

1999   Dr. Atkins publishes yet another revision.

recognized experts in food and nutrition, foodservice management, and wellness . . . We need the courage to perceive ourselves succeeding in new roles, to attract a diversity of people to dietetics, and to polish and practice marketing, management, leadership, and sales skills.[39]

Change is occurring rapidly in all areas of the dietetics profession—education, research, and practice. At an address to the American Dietetics Association in 2003, the Surgeon General of the United States, Richard Carmona, commended the professional association for its leadership in advancing healthcare quality through nutrition. One of his main priorities as Surgeon General was disease prevention. He stated that 7 out of 10 Americans who die each year die of a chronic disease, most of which are preventable by relatively simple steps: healthy eating, being active, and not smoking. Current efforts to encourage Americans to adopt healthy behaviors to prevent disease have not been successful. One of the reasons for this failure is low health literacy. **Health literacy** is an individual's ability to access, understand, and use health-related information and services to make appropriate health decisions. The inadequacy of nutrition education in medical schools is another concern, as 8 of the 10 leading diseases in the United States are linked to nutrition.[40]

The surgeon general challenged dietitians to make sure that their patients understand what they can do to stay healthy. He said:

Nutrition education is your business! Every single day you translate complex nutrition principles into an array of healthy eating options for the American public . . . your expertise is valued at the highest levels. Wherever you are—in clinics, hospitals, outpatient or long-term care settings, in sports, education or the restaurant and food industry—your work is tremendously important to the health and well being of Americans. And your work is becoming more and more important as we move towards a national prevention agenda. We need you—your passion, your expertise and your experience as nutrition professionals.[40]

A recent president of the Academy of Nutrition and Dietetics stated that trends toward preventive care and people's interest in achieving and maintaining an overall healthy lifestyle are two of the most dramatic developments affecting dietetics in the last two decades. To best adapt to these positive changes, she advised dietitians to sharpen their professional skills, gain deeper understanding of the unique needs of diverse populations, use critical-thinking skills to solve the difficult problems facing their communities, and seek opportunities for leadership.[41]

The priority areas at this time are aging, child nutrition, healthcare reform, nutrigenomics, sustainability, medical nutritional therapy, nutritional monitoring, nutrition research, obesity, and state government issues related to dietetics. Other food and nutrition areas of current importance are hunger, food insecurity, HIV/AIDS, food safety, allied health, and physical activity.

On January 1, 2012 the American Dietetic Association officially became the Academy of Nutrition and Dietetics. The name change was enacted to better reflect the strong science background and academic expertise of members, the academy's mission, vision, philosophy, and values.[42]

Summary

Although there is a long history of the relationship of food to health, the profession of dietetics is very young. Much of the progress in the profession has been made in the last 100 years (**Table 1–2**). Advances in scientific research, legislation, social and economic factors, military conflicts, and the leadership of some dynamic and dedicated dietitians have contributed to the advancement of the profession.

"Remember the 'old girls,' as they made it possible for us to work for our dream." This statement was made by Marion Mason, PhD, RD, Ruby Winslow Professor of Nutrition, Emerita, at Simmons College in Boston, in an address to the Massachusetts Dietetic Association.[43] It was Lulu Graves, the first president of the ADA, who first sounded the call for teamwork between physicians and dietitians. "The future of dietetics is assured. It is the privilege of those of us who are now in the work to conduct it along such lines that, in the not very distant future, it will be recognized as part of the medical team."[44] That time has arrived!

The increasing diversity of the profession through the years has created the need to broaden the focus of this goal. The ADA was founded at a time when most dietitians worked in acute-care hospitals. Just 26% of dietitians and 33% of dietetic technicians are now employed in this setting.[45] At the beginning of the twenty-first century, Lulu Graves's quote could be modified to read: It is the privilege of those of us who are now in the work to

TABLE 1–2

A Timeline of Selected Milestones in Dietetic History

2500 B.C.	Avoidance of onions is the first known dietary prescription.
1500 B.C.	Nutrient deficiency disease, scurvy, is described.
100 B.C.	Apicius's *De re Culinaria* is the first known cookbook.
1061	Ben Cao Tu Jing tests efficacy of ginseng.
1087	William the Conqueror goes on liquid diet to lose weight.
1123	St. Bartholomew's Hospital, London, is founded.
1478	*De re Medicina* is published in Florence, Italy. Diet becomes part of medical practice.
1480	First cookbook is printed.
1731	First hospital in United States is built in Philadelphia, Pennsylvania.
1747	James Lind conducts clinical trial on scurvy patients.
1792	Lavoisier outlines process of the "physiology of nutrition."
1811	Lord Byron uses vinegar to lose weight.
1854	Florence Nightingale uses nutrition to reduce death rate of soldiers.
1864	William Banting's bestseller touts high-protein diet for weight loss.
1872	Iowa Agricultural School offers courses in cookery.
1876	Dr. John Harvey Kellogg develops toasted flakes and granola.
1877	Kansas State offers course in household chemistry, and the American Medical Association forms committee on dietetics.
1878	Sarah Tyson Rorer opens Philadelphia Cooking School.
1884	Kanehiro Takaki adds milk and vegetables to Japanese sailors' diet of polished rice in order to cure beriberi.
1889	Christiaan Eijkman proposes nutritional hypothesis for beriberi.
1896	USDA publishes first food composition tables.
1898	Horace Fletcher proposes "Fletcherizing" for weight loss.
1899	The title of *dietitian* is defined.
1903	New York Department of Charities offers the first dietetic internship.
1907	William Fletcher conducts randomized trial on cause of beriberi.
1912	Casimir Funk isolates "vitamins" and suggests that dietary deficiencies of vitamins cause beriberi, rickets, pellagra, sprue, and other diseases.
1914	World War I boosts impetus for nutrition research.
1917	The American Dietetic Association is founded.
1920	Title *nutritionist* first appears, and the Maternity and Infancy Act allows states to employ nutritionists.
1921	Insulin is discovered.
1930	Spelling of *dietitian* is agreed upon.
1933	Robert R. Williams synthesizes and names vitamin B_1.
1935	Title V of the Social Security Act—federal funding for nutrition positions.
1938	Conrad Elvehjem identifies niacin as the missing nutrient causing pellagra.
1939	World War II contributes to public recognition of dietitians.
1946	National School Lunch Act expands dietetics to include school lunches.
1947	First national dieting group is founded—TOPS.
1960	Overeaters Anonymous is founded.

1961	Weight Watchers is founded.
1968	Expanded food and nutrition education programs for low-income families.
1969	Registration of dietitians is begun.
1972	Women, Infants, and Children Program (WIC) is started.
1975	Nutrition education program added to WIC.
1977	Food and Agriculture Act includes a nutrition education component.
1983	Certification of dietetic technicians is begun.
1993	Specialty board certification for RDs is started.
1999	Registration exams first administered by computer.
2010	2009 Code of Ethics for the Profession of Dietetics goes into effect.
2012	American Dietetic Association becomes the Academy of Nutrition and Dietetics.

conduct it along such lines that, in the not very distant future, it will be recognized as the best source for nutrition information and the professionals as those best trained to help consumers make individualized food choices. This comprehensive goal is exemplified in the words inscribed on the Academy of Nutrition and Dietetics seal, adopted in 1940, *Quam Plurimis Prodesse*—"to benefit as many as possible."

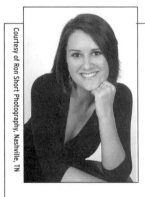

Courtesy of Ron Short Photography, Nashville, TN

Profile of a Professional

Sarah Vaughn, RD, LDN

Director/Nutrition Consultant
Nashville Fire Department and Metropolitan Nashville
    Police Department
Wellness Initiative, Nashville, Tennessee

Education:
BS in Nutrition, University of Tennessee, Knoxville, Tennessee
Dietetic Internship, Vanderbilt University Medical Center,
    Nashville, Tennessee

Where did you first hear about dietetics and decide to become a registered dietitian?
I first heard about dietetics from my school advisor as well as my mother, who would tell you that I was always very interested in the topic of nutrition. During my freshman year in college, I decided to follow my passions. I loved to cook, loved all topics on nutrition/wellness, and enjoyed helping others. Dietetics was a way to bring all of these things together. I knew then this was the profession for me!

What was your route to registration?
I completed the Didactic Program in Dietetics at the University of Tennessee in Knoxville and then a dietetic internship at Vanderbilt University Medical Center in Nashville, Tennessee.

What has been your career path in dietetics and what are you doing now?
After my dietetic internship, I was contacted by a preceptor of mine about initiating a new wellness program for Nashville's public safety. As an entry-level RD, I had the opportunity to shape the position of the registered dietitian as well as promote

the first wellness program for the Nashville Fire Department and the Metropolitan Nashville Police Department. Currently, I am director and nutrition consultant for the program. It is a rewarding experience!

Are you involved in any professional organizations?
I've been secretary of the Nashville District Dietetic Association, Public Policy Coordinator for the Tennessee Dietetic Association, a volunteer for the Academy of Nutrition and Dietetics Weight Management Dietetic Practice Group newsletter-editing team, and a member of the Tennessee Public Health Association.

Have you received any honors or awards?
I was honored to be featured on the cover and in the lead article of the summer 2009 issue of what was then known as the *ADA Times*. The article featured my work with firefighters and public safety.

Is teamwork important to you in your position?
Teamwork is very important to my current position. As a member of the wellness team, I communicate with the Occupational Health and Wellness staff, including the Civil Service Medical Examiner, the nurse practitioner and nursing staff, and the exercise physiologist. Together, as a team, we are able to provide excellent care and information for our public safety population. Not only am I constantly involved in team projects with my coworkers in the wellness program, but I am also involved in various projects for the Metro Public Health Department. There are always individuals in your workplace with knowledge and skills who can enable you, as the RD, to strengthen your job, program, and ways of communicating messages to the public.

What excites you about dietetics and the future of our profession?
What excites me about dietetics are the endless possibilities of where registered dietitians can work and how they can help communities with their nutrition expertise. There is a new wave of technology that RDs can utilize to promote their services and nutrition information. It is fascinating to watch the evolution of the dietetics profession. I look forward to seeing the role of the registered dietitian be recognized as a major component in the overall health and well-being of individuals.

What words of wisdom do you have for future dietetics professionals?
Always be open for new and exciting opportunities in your career. Don't be afraid to use your creativity and knowledge as a registered dietitian to implement a new idea and continue to build your skills to better serve your clients and/or community. Take your passion, whatever drives you, and make nutrition your career path.

Suggested Activities

1. Search the Internet to find additional contributions Lavoisier made to the practice of dietetics, specifically in the areas of food hygiene and hospital sanitation.

2. The James Lind Library has been created to introduce people to the characteristics of fair tests of medical treatments. Visit the Library's website (www.jameslindlibrary.org) to find out the characteristics of a "fair test." Compare your findings to the definition of the scientific method.

3. Use the Internet to research the history of pellagra. When was it determined that pellagra was a vitamin-deficiency disease? Who made this discovery? Which vitamin was missing from the diets of those who became ill with pellagra? Why was this vitamin not present in their diet?

4. What are the most recent developments within the dietetics profession? Visit the website of the Academy of Nutrition and Dietetics (www .eatright.org) to read the latest news. Read the press release announcing the name change. Discuss the reasons for the name change.

5. How does dietetic practice differ in other countries? Do an Internet search to compare international dietetic associations.

6. Many of the weight-loss regimens listed in this chapter would be considered "quackery." Visit www.dietetics.com and click the "Antiquackery" link to see what is being done today to combat such practices.

7. Read one of the autobiographies in *Legends and Legacies* (C. E. Vickery and N. Cotugna, Kendall/Hunt Publishing, 1990) and give an oral report to your class.

8. Secure a very old book on health or cooking from a library or used bookstore. Compare its content to present-day beliefs and practices.

9. Interview a 50-year member of the profession to obtain a personal history of changes that have occurred in the dietetics profession.

10. Read a journal article chronicling the history of dietetic practice during World War I or II. Two examples are:

   - Hodges PA. Perspective on history: military dietetics in Europe during World War I. *J Am Diet Assoc.* 1993;93:897–900.
   - Hodges PA. Perspective on history: military dietetics in the Philippines during World War II. *J Am Diet Assoc.* 1992;92:840–843.

Selected Websites

- www.chemheritage.org—The Chemical Heritage Foundation fosters an understanding of chemistry's impact on society.
- www.eatright.org—The Academy of Nutrition and Dietetics is the world's largest organization of food and nutrition professionals.
- www.jameslindlibrary.org—The James Lind Library seeks to help people understand the fair tests of treatments in health care.
- www.prbm.com—The Philadelphia Rare Books and Manuscripts Company offers a variety of old and rare nutrition- and health-related books.

Suggested Readings

Banting FG, Best CH, Collip JB, Campbell WR, Fletcher AA. Pancreatic extracts in the treatment of diabetes mellitus. *Can Med Assoc J.* 1922;12:141–146.

Fletcher W. Rice and beri-beri: Preliminary report on an experiment conducted in the Kuala Lumpur Insane Asylum. *Lancet.* 1907;1:1776–1779.

Fraser L. *Losing It: America's Obsession with Weight and the Industry That Feeds on It.* New York: EP Dutton; 1997.

Funk C. *The Vitamines.* Authorized translation from 2nd German ed. By Dubin HE. Baltimore: Williams & Wilkins; 1922.

Mestel R. Round and round we go. *Los Angeles Times,* December 29, 2003, Section F, p. 1.

Stearns P. *Fat History.* New York: New York University Press; 2002.

Vickery C, Cotugna N. *Legends and Legacies.* Dubuque, IA: Kendall/Hunt Publishing; 1990.

References

1. Why study history? Radford University Department of History website. http://www .radford.edu/content/chbs/home/history/why-history.html. Accessed April 13, 2010.

2. Jastrow, M. *The Civilization of Babylonia and Assyria*. Philadelphia: JB Lippincott; 1915.

3. *The Bible* (revised standard version), Judges 13:14. New York: Collins; 1971.

4. *The Bible* (revised standard version), Daniel 1:5–16. New York: Collins; 1971.

5. Huskey RJ. A simple experiment on scurvy. Available at: http://www.ca-biomed.org/csbr /pdf/nut.pdf. Accessed April 13, 2010.

6. Gove PB, ed. *Webster's Third New International Dictionary*. Springfield, MA: G & C Merriam; 1971.

7. Barber MI, ed. *History of the American Dietetic Association (1917–1959)*. Philadelphia: JB Lippincott; 1959.

8. Vehling JD, trans. *Apicius: Cooking and Dining in Imperial Rome*. Chicago: Walter M. Hill; 1936.

9. Whang J. Chinese traditional food therapy. *J Am Diet Assoc*. 1981;78:55–57.

10. Durant W. *Our Oriental Heritage*. New York: Simon & Schuster; 1935.

11. Garrison FH. *An Introduction to the History of Medicine*, 4th ed. Philadelphia: WB Saunders; 1967.

12. Cao Tu Jing B. *Atlas of Materia Medica*. Collected and edited by Shang Z. Anhui Science and Technology Press (in Chinese); 1994.

13. Isch C. A history of hospital fare. In: Beeuwkes AM, Todhunter EN, Weigley ES, eds. *Essays on the History of Nutrition and Dietetics*. Chicago: The American Dietetic Association; 1967.

14. De Honesta Voluptate. In: Whitcomb M, ed. *Literary Source Book of the Italian Renaissance*. Philadelphia; 1900.

15. Swartz H. *Never Satisfied*. New York: Free Press; 1986.

16. The American Dietetic Association Study Commission on Dietetics. *A New Look at the Profession of Dietetics*. Chicago: The American Dietetic Association; 1984.

17. Needham J. Clerks and craftsmen in China and the West. In: *Lectures and Addresses on the History of Science and Technology*. Cambridge, MA: Cambridge University Press; 1970.

18. Rabenn WB. Hospital diets in eighteenth century England. In: Beeuwkes AM, Todhunter EN, Weigley ES, eds. *Essays on the History of Nutrition and Dietetics*. Chicago: The American Dietetic Association; 1967.

19. Cooper LF. Florence Nightingale's contribution to dietetics. In: Beeuwkes AM, Todhunter EN, Weigley ES, eds. *Essays on the History of Nutrition and Dietetics*. Chicago: The American Dietetic Association; 1967.

20. Gilson HE. Some historical notes on the development of diet therapy. In: Beeuwkes AM, Todhunter EN, Weigley ES, eds. *Essays on the History of Nutrition and Dietetics*. Chicago: The American Dietetic Association; 1967.

21. Cooper LF. The dietitian and her profession. *J Am Diet Assoc*. 1938;4:751–758.

22. Rorer ST. Early dietetics. *J Am Diet Assoc*. 1934;x:289.

23. Rorer ST. Feeding the sick. *Household News*. 1893;1:69. Rorer ST. How to design a kitchen. *Household News*. 1894;2:17. Rorer ST. Answers to inquiries. *Household News*. 1893;1:13.

24. Weigley ES. Sarah Tyson Rorer. First American dietitian? *J Am Diet Assoc*. 1980;77:11–15.

25. Jikei University School of Medicine. Founding Spirit—Patient-Centered Medical Care. Available at: http://www.jikei.ac.jp/outline/en_history2.html. Accessed January 15, 2004.

26. Vandenbroucke JP. The contribution of William Fletcher's 1907 report to finding a cause and cure for beriberi. The James Lind Library. Available at: http://www.jameslindlibrary .org/illustrating/articles/the-contribution-of-william-fletchers-1907-report-to-finding-a. Accessed January 13, 2004.

27. Atwater WO, Bryant AF. *The Chemical Composition of American Food Materials*. U.S. Department of Agriculture Bulletin No. 28. Washington, DC: U.S. Government Printing Office; 1896.

28. Corbett FR. The training of dietitians for hospitals. *J Home Econ.* 1909;1:62.

29. Funk C. The etiology of the deficiency diseases. *J State Med.* 1912;341–368.

30. Egan M. Public health nutrition services: issues today and tomorrow. *J Am Diet Assoc.* 1980;77:423.

31. Burnett J. *Plenty and Want: A Social History of Diet in England from 1815 to the Present Day.* London: Nelson; 1966.

32. Baylor University. History of Military Dietitians. Available at: http://www.baylor.edu /graduate/nutrition/index.php?id=68073. Accessed December 26, 2009.

33. Minot GR, Murphy WP. Treatment of pernicious anaemia by a special diet. *J Am Diet Assoc.* 1926;87:470–476.

34. Eliot MM, Heseltine MM. Nutrition in maternal and child health programs. *Nutrition Review.* 1947:533–535.

35. Bray GA. Nutrition in the Humphrey tradition. *J Am Diet Assoc.* 1979;75:116–121.

36. Cross AT. USDA's strategies for the 80s: nutrition education. *J Am Diet Assoc.* 1980;76:333–337.

37. Ritchie Hartwick, AM. Army Medical Specialist Corps in Vietnam. Available at: http:// www.vietnamwomensmemorial.org/pdf/ahartwick.pdf. Accessed December 22, 2009.

38. ADA testifies in favor of improving USDA domestic feeding programs. *ADA Courier.* 1993;32:2.

39. Calvert-Finn S, Rinke W. Probing the envelope of dietetics by transforming challenges into opportunities. *J Am Diet Assoc.* 1980;89:1441–1443.

40. Carmona RH. Remarks at ADA's 2003 Food & Nutrition Conference and Expo, San Antonio, TX, October 27, 2003.

41. Smith Edge, M. Remarks at ADA's 2003 Food & Nutrition Conference & Expo, San Antonio, TX, October 27, 2003.

42. Academy of Nutrition and Dietetics. Press Release: American Dietetic Association Officially Becomes the Academy of Nutrition and Dietetics. Available at: http://www .eatright.org. Accessed January 3, 2012.

43. Fitz PA. President's page: About 80 years ago . . . *J Am Diet Assoc.* 1997;97:1160–1161.

44. Cassell JA. *Carry the Flame: The History of the American Dietetic Association.* Chicago: The American Dietetic Association; 1990.

45. The American Dietetic Association. *2009 Dietetics Compensation & Benefits Survey of the Dietetics Profession.* Chicago: The American Dietetic Association; 2010.

The Present

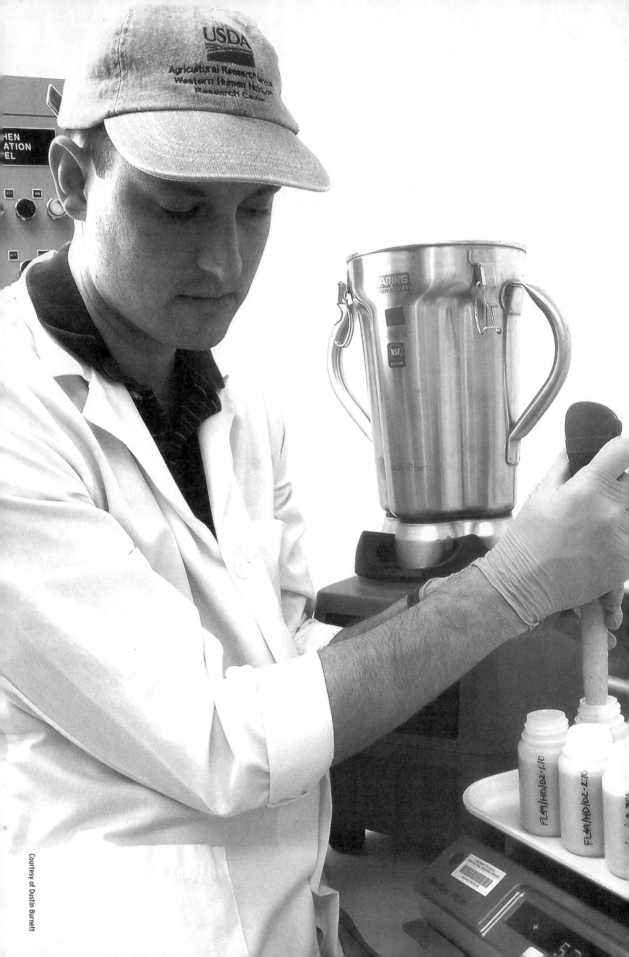

The Dietetics Profession

"To benefit as many as possible", appeared on the seal of the American Dietetic Association (and is still in use today on the seal of the Academy of Nutrition and Dietetics). It is an even more relevant goal of the profession today than it was in 1940 when it was first adopted. The scope of professional practice is continuously widening, and the knowledge base of nutrition is deepening. Since that first meeting in Cleveland in 1917, the Academy of Nutrition and Dietetics has grown to be the largest food and nutrition organization in the world. This growth has occurred because of members who are willing to seize and/or create opportunities and who have solid educational foundations that are diverse enough to allow practice in a myriad of areas.

What is dietetics? What makes it a profession? Who are today's dietitians? Where do they work, and what do they do? What kind of compensation and benefits do they enjoy in their positions, and what are some of the issues facing the profession today? These are the questions that are addressed in this chapter (**Figure 2–1**).

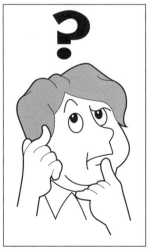

FIGURE 2–1 Just what is dietetics?

What Is Dietetics?

At the center of the professional association seal, adopted in 1940, are images representing the three main characteristics of the profession: a balance, representing science as the foundation of dietetics; a caduceus, representing the close relationship between dietetics and medicine; and a cooking vessel, representing cooking and food preparation. Surrounding this is a shaft of wheat, representing bread as the staff of life; acanthus leaves, representing growth and life, and a cornucopia, representing an abundant food supply.

Consider the following definitions of *dietetics*:

- "The scientific study of food preparation and intake."[1]
- "The science of applying nutritional principles to the planning and preparation of foods and regulation of the diet in relation to both health and disease."[2]

These definitions are woefully inadequate for what dietetics has grown to become. The basis of dietetics is the firm belief that optimal nutrition is essential for the health and well-being of every person. This is why dietetics is an integral component of the healthcare field. A team effort by doctors, nurses, and dietitians is usually necessary to return a patient to health. However, it is possible that no other profession offers such a diversity of opportunities outside of the traditional healthcare arena as the field of dietetics. Early dietetic practitioners were usually found in an institutional kitchen—for which the dictionary definitions would have been adequate. Today, dietitians can be found almost anywhere. For this reason, a recent survey of dietetics made use of a very broad definition of *dietetics*:

> A dietetics-related position is considered to be any position that requires or makes use of your education, training, and/or experience in dietetics or nutrition, including situations outside of "traditional" dietetics practice.[3]

What Is a Profession?

A general definition of a *profession* might be "an occupation for which preliminary training is intellectual in character, involving knowledge and learning as distinguished from mere skill, which is pursued largely for others and not merely for oneself and in which financial return is not an accepted measure of success."[4]

The Goals Committee of the Academy of Nutrition and Dietetics interprets a profession as a calling requiring the following:

- Specialized knowledge and often long and intensive preparation
- Maintenance, by force of organization or concerted opinion, of high standards of achievement and conduct
- Instruction in skills and methods as well as scientific, historical, or scholarly principles underlying such skills and methods
- Commitment of its members to continued study
- A kind of work that has as its primary purpose the rendering of a public service[5]

A professional is one who represents or belongs to a profession.

How Is Dietetics a Profession?

Five main characteristics of dietetic practice qualify it for professional status:

1. A specialized body of knowledge
2. Specialized services rendered to society
3. An obligation for service to the client that overrides personal considerations
4. Concern for competence and honor among the practitioners
5. An obligation to continuing education, research, and sharing of knowledge for the common good[6]

What Is a Registered Dietitian?

A dietitian has been defined as "a professional person who is a translator of the science and art of foods, nutrition, and dietetics in the service of people—whether individually or in families or larger groups; healthy or sick; and at all stages of the life cycle."[6]

Some titles need to be clarified at this point: *dietitian, registered dietitian, nutritionist, licensed dietitian,* and *dietetic technician* (**Figure 2–2**). The title of dietitian usually implies a registered dietitian, or RD. An RD has completed the required academic training and supervised practice program (described in Chapters 5 and 6) and has successfully passed the national credentialing exam. There are no such requirements for the use of the title "nutritionist"; the term has no standards of education or training. This means that anyone can use the title nutritionist with little or no training in the field—and many do. However, some registered dietitians choose to use the title nutritionist, particularly those working in public health. A few states restrict the use of these titles unless the person has completed a certain amount of education and training.[7]

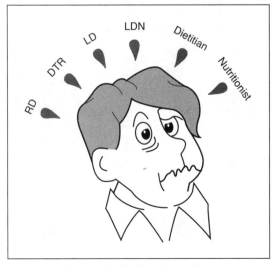

FIGURE 2–2 Titles used in the dietetics profession.

Many states have regulatory laws that either require or permit dietitians to be licensed. A licensed dietitian or licensed dietitian/nutritionist (LD or LDN) is a person who has been licensed by a state to ensure competence. State requirements for licensure are frequently met through the same education, training, and national exam required for RDs.[7]

Registered dietitian (RD) is a nationally recognized title for a nutrition expert. This title reflects the high level of entry-level education and training and the continuing education required to achieve and maintain RD status. In addition, some RDs have achieved additional certification in specialized areas of practice, such as pediatric nutrition (CSP, Board Certified Specialist in Pediatric Nutrition), renal nutrition (CSR, Board Certified Specialist in Renal Nutrition), sports nutrition (CSSD, Board Certified Specialist in Sports Dietetics), gerontologic nutrition (CSG, Board Certified Specialist in Gerontological Nutrition), and oncology nutrition (CSO, Board Certified Specialist in Oncology Nutrition).[7]

The title dietetic technician, like dietitian, implies that the person is a registered dietetic technician (DTR) (**Figure 2–3**). DTRs are trained in food and nutrition and are an integral part of healthcare and foodservice management teams. Like RDs, DTRs must complete an academic program and a supervised practice experience and must pass a national written exam in order to use the title.[7]

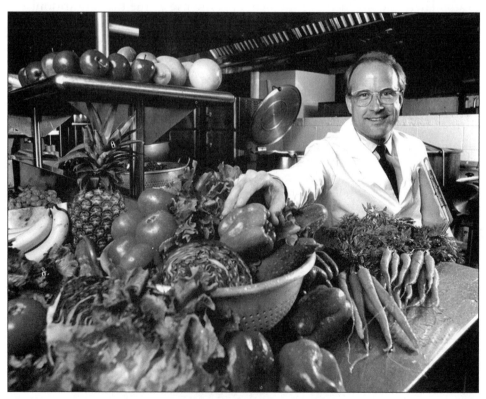

FIGURE 2–3 A registered dietetic technician (DTR) at work.
Courtesy of the Academy of Nutrition and Dietetics

From the Academy of Nutrition and Dietetics Definition of Terms:

The Commission on Dietetic Registration defines the Registered Dietitian (RD) as an individual who has met current minimum (Baccalaureate) academic requirements with successful completion of both specified didactic education and supervised-practice experiences through programs accredited by The Accreditation Council for Education in Nutrition and Dietetics (ACEND) of the Academy of Nutrition and Dietetics and who has successfully completed the Registration Examination for Dietitians. To maintain the RD credential, the RD must comply with the Professional Development Portfolio (PDP) recertification requirements (accrue 75 units of approved continuing professional education every five years).[8]

The Commission on Dietetic Registration defines the Dietetic Technician, Registered (DTR) as an individual who has met current minimum requirements through one of three routes: (1) Successful completion of a minimum of an Associate degree and Dietetic Technician Program through a program accredited by Accreditation Council for Education in Nutrition and Dietetics (ACEND) of The Academy of Nutrition and Dietetics (Academy). (2) Successful completion of a Baccalaureate degree; met current academic requirements (Didactic Program in Dietetics) as accredited by ACEND of the Academy; successfully completed a supervised practice program under the auspices of a Dietetic Technician Program as accredited by ACEND. (3) Completed a minimum of a Baccalaureate degree; successfully completed a Didactic Program in Dietetics as accredited by ACEND of the Academy. In all three routes, the individual must successfully complete the Registration Examination for Dietetic Technicians. To maintain the DTR credential, the DTR must comply with the Professional Development Portfolio (PDP) recertification requirements (accrue 50 hours of approved continuing professional education every five years).[8]

Dietetic practice is based on the application of principles derived from the integration of knowledge from many disciplines. Successful dietetic practitioners then apply skills and attitudes to translate this knowledge in order to achieve and maintain the health of people. **Figure 2–4** is a graphic depiction of the knowledge areas, skills, and attitudes essential for successful dietetic practice.

Who Are Dietitians?

A recent survey, which included a sample of 9,556 members of the Academy of Nutrition and Dietetics, found that 96% of dietetic practitioners are female, with a median age of 47. The field is predominantly white; 8% of respondents indicated a race other than white and 3% identified themselves as Hispanic. The median number of years of work experience was 17. Almost all RDs hold bachelor's degrees, with 46% having a master's degree and 4% a doctorate. Seventy-four percent of RDs are members of the Academy of Nutrition and Dietetics, 47% have a state license, and 19% hold one or more specialty certifications.[3]

Twenty-eight percent of DTRs hold a bachelor's degree or higher, and 43% are members of the Academy of Nutrition and Dietetics. Eight percent of DTRs hold a state license, and 10% hold one or more specialty certifications.[3]

Where Do Dietitians Work and What Do They Do?

Dietitians seem to work everywhere and do everything. More specifically, the professional association's 2009 Compensation and Benefit Survey found that the most common employment setting is the hospital: 26% of dietitians and 33% of DTRs work in a hospital setting. Ten percent of RDs and 32% of

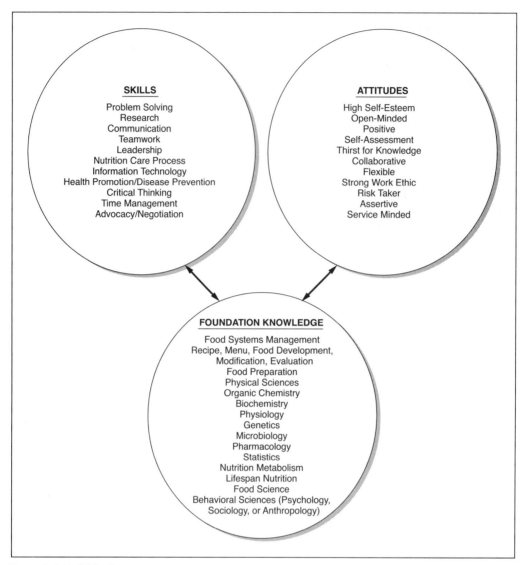

SKILLS

Problem Solving
Research
Communication
Teamwork
Leadership
Nutrition Care Process
Information Technology
Health Promotion/Disease Prevention
Critical Thinking
Time Management
Advocacy/Negotiation

ATTITUDES

High Self-Esteem
Open-Minded
Positive
Self-Assessment
Thirst for Knowledge
Collaborative
Flexible
Strong Work Ethic
Risk Taker
Assertive
Service Minded

FOUNDATION KNOWLEDGE

Food Systems Management
Recipe, Menu, Food Development,
Modification, Evaluation
Food Preparation
Physical Sciences
Organic Chemistry
Biochemistry
Physiology
Genetics
Microbiology
Pharmacology
Statistics
Nutrition Metabolism
Lifespan Nutrition
Food Science
Behavioral Sciences (Psychology,
Sociology, or Anthropology)

FIGURE 2–4 Model for dietetic practice.

DTRs work in an extended-care facility, 13% of RDs and 2% of DTRs work in a clinic or ambulatory care center, and 13% of both RDs and DTRs work in a community or public health program. A little more than one in five dietetic practitioners (21%) is not currently employed. The remaining practitioners work in a wide variety of other settings (**Figure 2–5**). Ten percent are self-employed (primarily RDs), 40% work for a nonprofit firm, 30% for a for-profit company, and 19% for the government.[3]

Dietetic practice can be divided into seven key areas: clinical—acute care/inpatient, clinical—ambulatory care, clinical—long-term care, food and nutrition management, community, consultation and business, and education and research. Within these seven areas, 40 different job titles account for 80% of all dietetic employment.[9] The percentage breakdown for those working in these seven practice areas is shown in **Table 2–1**.

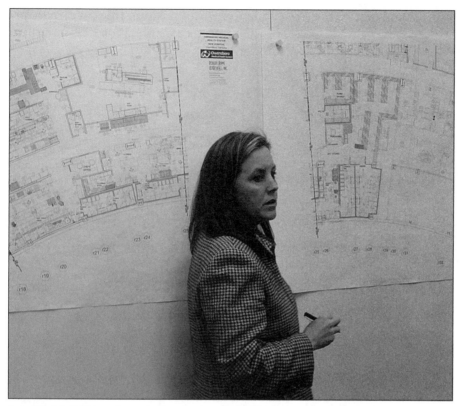

FIGURE 2–5 A dietitian who works for a foodservice facility design company.
Courtesy of Christine Guyott, RD

TABLE 2-1

Percentage of Dietitians in the Seven Practice Areas in the Field of Dietetics

Practice Area	RDs	DTRs
Clinical nutrition acute care/inpatient	30%	39%
Clinical nutrition ambulatory care	17%	1%
Clinical nutrition long-term care	9%	17%
Food and nutrition management	12%	19%
Community	11%	10%
Consultation and business	8%	2%
Education and research	7%	2%

DTRs, registered dietetic technicians; RDs, registered dietitians.

Data from: American Dietetic Association. 2009 Compensation and Benefits Survey of the American Dietetic Association. Chicago: The American Dietetic Association; 2010.

The following are the most commonly held position titles in dietetic practice (note that the percentages of the top eight positions for RDs and the top five for DTRs are given in parentheses):

Clinical—Acute Care/Inpatient

Dietetic technician, clinical (36%)

Clinical dietitian (16%)

Clinical dietitian, specialist—cardiac

Clinical dietitian, specialist—diabetes

Clinical dietitian, specialist—oncology

Clinical dietitian, specialist—renal

Clinical dietitian, specialist—other

Pediatric/neonatal dietitian

Nutrition support dietitian

Clinical—Ambulatory Care

Outpatient dietitian, general (4%)

Outpatient dietitian, specialist—cardiac rehabilitation

Outpatient dietitian, specialist—diabetes (5%)

Outpatient dietitian, specialist—pediatrics

Outpatient dietitian, specialist—renal (4%)

Outpatient dietitian, specialist—weight management

Outpatient dietitian, specialist—other

Home-care dietitian

Clinical—Long-Term Care

Clinical dietitian, long-term care (9%)

Dietetic technician, long-term care (13%)

Food and Nutrition Management

Executive-level professional

Administrative dietitian—patient care

Assistant director of foodservices

Clinical nutrition manager

Director of food and nutrition services (4% of RDs and 5% of DTRs)

School foodservice director

Dietetic technician, foodservice management (9%)

Community

Women, Infants, and Children (WIC) nutritionist (5% of RDs and 8% of DTRs)

Cooperative extension educator/specialist

Corrections dietitian

Public health nutritionist

School/child care nutritionist

Nutrition coordinator for Head Start program

Nutritionist for food bank or assistance program

Consultation and Business

Private practice dietitian—patient/client nutrition care (2%)

Consultant—communications

Sales representative

Consultant—community and/or corporate programs

Public relations and/or marketing professional

Corporate account manager

Corporate dietitian

Director of nutrition

Manager of nutrition communications

Research and development nutritionist

Education and Research

Instructor/lecturer

Assistant or associate professor

Chair, Department of Nutrition and Food Science

Clinical research dietitian

Administrator, higher education

Didactic program director

Dietetic internship director

Professor[3]

In summary, most RDs are found in the following settings:

- **Hospitals, health maintenance organizations (HMOs), and other health-care facilities.** RDs educate patients about nutrition and administer medical nutrition therapy (MNT) as part of the healthcare team. They also manage the foodservice operation, where they oversee everything from food purchasing and preparation to managing the staff (**Figure 2–6**).

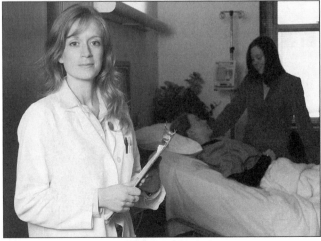

FIGURE 2–6 A clinical dietitian.
Courtesy of the Academy of Nutrition and Dietetics

- **Schools, day care centers, and correctional facilities.** RDs manage the foodservice operations, including planning menus, purchasing food, supervising preparation, and directing the staff (**Figure 2–7**).
- **Sports nutrition and corporate wellness programs.** RDs educate clients about the connections among food, fitness, and health (**Figure 2–8**).
- **Food- and nutrition-related businesses and industries.** RDs work in communications, consumer affairs, public relations, marketing, and product development.

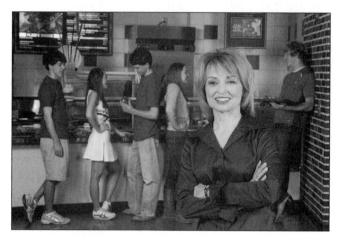

FIGURE 2–7 A dietitian who works in school foodservice.
Courtesy of the Academy of Nutrition and Dietetics

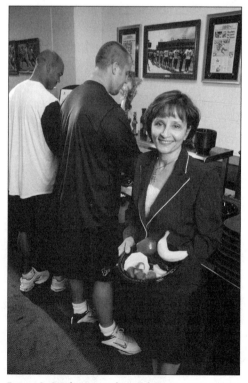

FIGURE 2–8 A dietitian who works in sports nutrition.
Courtesy of the Academy of Nutrition and Dietetics

- **Private practice.** RDs work under contract with healthcare or food companies or in their own business. RDs provide services to restaurant and foodservice managers, food vendors and distributors, athletes, nursing home residents, and company employees.
- **Community and public health settings.** RDs teach, monitor, advise, and help the public to improve their quality of life through the promotion of healthy eating habits.
- **Universities and medical centers.** RDs teach physicians, nurses, dietetics students and interns, and others the science of food and nutrition.
- **Research facilities.** RDs direct and collaborate on experimental research to answer critical questions at food and pharmaceutical companies, universities, and hospitals.[10]

DTRs may also be found working independently or in teams with RDs in a variety of work settings, including health care, business and industry, public health, foodservice, and research. DTRs most commonly work in:

- **Hospitals, HMOs, clinics, nursing homes, retirement centers, hospices, home healthcare agencies, and research facilities.** DTRs treat and prevent disease and administer MNT as an important part of the healthcare team.
- **Schools, day care centers, correctional facilities, restaurants, healthcare facilities, corporations, and hospitals.** DTRs manage foodservice operations, including food purchasing and preparation, supervising employees, and teaching nutrition classes (**Figure 2–9**).

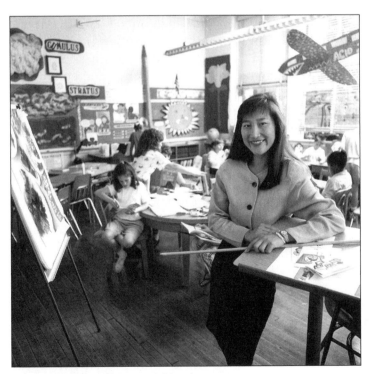

FIGURE 2–9 A DTR teaching a nutrition class.
Courtesy of the Academy of Nutrition and Dietetics

- **WIC programs, public health agencies, Meals on Wheels, and community health programs.** DTRs develop and teach nutrition classes for the public.
- **Health clubs, weight-management clinics, and community wellness centers.** DTRs educate clients about the connections among food, fitness, and health.
- **Food companies, contract food management companies, food vendors, and food distribution companies.** DTRs develop menus, oversee food-service sanitation and food safety, and prepare food labeling information and nutrient analysis.[10]

What Is the Salary Range for RDs and DTRs?

As is true for most professions, the salary range and fees charged vary by region of the country, employment setting, scope of responsibility, and supply and demand for RDs. According to the professional association's 2009 Compensation and Benefits Survey, the median annual income in the United States for dietitians who have been working at least one year is $58,000, and for DTRs who have been working in a position for at least one year it is $40,000.[3]

The statistics generated by the survey show that the dietitian's salary increases as the number of years in the field increases, as the number of years in the position increases, as higher graduate degrees are held, as the level and scope of responsibility increase, as the size of the budget that is managed increases, as the size of the employing organization increases, and as the number of people being supervised increases.[3]

Two other factors have an influence on salary—the area of practice and the area of the country. The highest-paying practice areas are food and nutrition management, consultation and business, and education and research. The lowest-paying areas are in clinical and community nutrition practice. According to the 2009 survey, the highest salaries were found in Washington, DC, California, Delaware, Maryland, and Utah. The top-paying metropolitan areas were:

- Washington, DC
- San Francisco, California
- Riverside/San Bernardino, California
- Los Angeles/Long Beach, California
- Sacramento, California
- Chicago, Illinois
- Atlanta, Georgia
- Miami, Florida
- San Antonio, Texas
- Boston, Massachusetts
- Kansas City, Missouri[3]

The states with members reporting the lowest salaries were South Carolina, Mississippi, Iowa, Kentucky, and West Virginia. Metropolitan

TABLE 2-2

Benefits Offered to Dietetics Professionals

Benefit	Employers' Offering (%)
Paid vacation, personal time off	82
Paid holidays	73
Paid sick days	71
Medical insurance, group plan or savings account	83
Dental insurance or group plan	78
Prescription drug benefit	71
Vision insurance or group plan	67
Life insurance	73
Disability insurance (long and/or short term)	64
Defined contribution retirement plan	66
Defined benefit retirement plan (pension)	38
Stock options	7
Profit sharing	7
Funding for professional development	50
Professional society dues	26
College tuition assistance	36
Employee assistance or wellness program	51
Comp time or flex time	32
Fitness benefit	39
Extended and/or paid parental leave	25
On-site child care or allowance	11
Telecommuting	9

Data from: American Dietetic Association. 2009 Compensation and Benefits Survey of the American Dietetic Association. Chicago: The American Dietetic Association; 2010.

areas with the lowest compensation were Milwaukee, Wisconsin; Nashville, Tennessee; Phoenix, Arizona; and St. Louis, Missouri.[3]

In addition to pay, fringe benefits are an important employment consideration. When compared with benefits of other professional technical employees in private industry, dietetic professionals' benefits are very favorable. The percentage of practitioners offered various benefits is shown in **Table 2–2**.

Specialty Areas and New Employment Opportunities

The dietetic profession is committed to helping people enjoy healthy lives. Therefore, five critical health areas confronting Americans have become priorities for the dietetics profession: (1) obesity and overweight, (2) aging, (3) complementary care and dietary supplements, (4) safe and nutritious food supply, and (5) human genome and genetics. Opportunities abound in these areas, as they do in the less traditional dietetic careers.[10]

As mentioned earlier, dietitians can be found working most anywhere. Consider the following nutrition-related employment opportunities that have not been mentioned previously:

Attorney

Author

Chef (**Figure 2–10**)

Educational representative for business

Extension service 4-H coordinator

Extension service home advisor

Food advertising consultant

Food analyst/technologist

Food broker

Food editor

Food journalist

Food photography specialist

Food quality assurance specialist

Food research and marketing specialist

Food science educator

Food scientist

Foodservice administrator for airline or cruise line

Foodservice equipment specialist

Food stylist

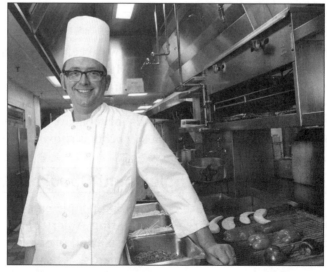

FIGURE 2–10 A dietitian who is a chef.
Courtesy of the Academy of Nutrition and Dietetics

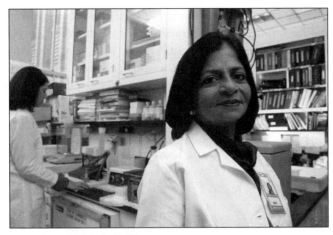

FIGURE 2–11 A research dietitian.
Courtesy of the Academy of Nutrition and Dietetics

Freelance writer

Home economist for food, equipment, or utility business

Job listing and placement service executive

Marketing specialist for a food or nutrition company

Media spokesperson

Motivational speaker

Peace Corps representative

Product development researcher

Publisher

Rehabilitation consultant

Research chemist (**Figure 2–11**)

Restaurant owner

Taste panel coordinator

Test kitchen scientist

This list is by no means exhaustive, but it shows the breadth of opportunities available to someone who has training in food and nutrition. The educational requirements for these positions vary from some college work to an advanced degree. Many do not require any credential, but some do. Some require additional training and/or education other than an advanced degree.

What Are Some of the Issues Facing Dietetic Practice?

This is an exciting time to be a nutrition professional. The knowledge that lifestyle choices, such as diet and exercise, can make a dramatic difference in quality of life is becoming more widespread. People are eager for information that can give them an edge in competitive sports, improve their appearance, make them feel better, and help them live longer, more productive lives. The knowledge that what we eat can dramatically affect our health will create a demand for those who can provide this information. Everybody needs us! Obesity is a worldwide health issue. A government-sponsored research study recently showed that the annual healthcare cost of obesity in the United States has doubled in less than a decade and may be as high as $147 billion a year.[11] Many people do not even know how to cook. In addition, the demand for quality control and reliability in the food industry is increasing.

Job growth in health care continues to be strong. The health-related professions have not suffered from the recent recession because of the aging of the U.S. population and increases in the number and type of available treatments. According to one expert, "While fast-food and customer-service may churn out a greater total volume of new jobs, those in health care are almost as plentiful and offer better pay, prospects, and benefits, plus the stability of a nearly recession-proof industry."[12] Over the next several years, job growth in health care is expected to be twice that of other industries. A number of factors account for this growth. The "graying of America" will create the need for more specialized medical care, home health care, and geriatric specialists. The increasing focus on wellness and preventive medicine by HMOs and by the public at large has also contributed to the expansion of the healthcare field.

The three fastest-growing career fields are health care, computers, and education. Dietetic practitioners are widely employed in each of these fields. Jobs that require a bachelor's degree or higher will grow at a rate almost double that of jobs that require only a high school diploma. The Bureau of Labor Statistics lists the employment of dietitians and nutritionists in 2008 as 60,300 and predicts that this number will increase by 9% from 2008 to 2018. This 9% increase is about the same as the average for all occupations requiring a college degree.[13–15]

Specific to the area of dietetics and nutrition, job growth will result from an increasing emphasis on disease prevention through improved dietary habits. The growing aging population will boost demand for nutritional counseling in hospitals, residential care facilities, schools, prisons, community health programs, and home healthcare agencies. The public's growing interest in nutrition, health education, and a prudent lifestyle will increase demand, especially in foodservice management. In addition, the increased prevalence and awareness of obesity and diabetes has resulted in Medicare coverage being expanded to include medical nutrition therapy for renal and diabetic patients. Dietitians specializing in these fields will benefit from this coverage.

The areas predicted to experience the fastest growth in job opportunities for dietetic practitioners are outpatient care facilities, physician offices, and foodservice management. Dietitians with specialized training, advanced degrees, and certifications beyond their state's minimum requirements will enjoy the best job opportunities. Those specializing in renal, diabetes, or gerontology will benefit from the growing number of people with diabetes and the aging of the population.

However, there may be some clouds on the otherwise rosy horizon of the healthcare industry. Cost-containment measures, such as budget cutting, downsizing, realignments, outsourcing, and mergers, may affect growth. Many predict that funding for Medicare programs will be reduced, forcing Medicare patients to pay for some home-care costs themselves. However, government surveys of job prospects indicate that healthcare reform will not shrink the workforce.

Negative factors specifically affecting job opportunities in dietetics and nutrition include the fact that some employers are substituting lower-paid workers to do nutrition-related work. Also, the demand for nutritional counseling is related to the patients' ability to pay, either out-of-pocket or through insurance reimbursement. Although the extent of insurance coverage for nutrition services has increased, it still varies widely. Hospitals and nursing care facilities still continue to employ large numbers of dietitians and dietetic technicians, but they also continue to contract with outside firms to run the foodservice operation and move medical nutrition therapy to outpatient departments.

Although dietetic practitioners are regarded as experts in nutrition, there is still some lack of recognition from the public. The American public has increased its knowledge and understanding of foods and nutrition, but misinformation still abounds. Popular magazines are full of attention-grabbing, but inaccurate, advice. Health food stores promote the sale of supposedly "super nutrients" to the tune of billions of dollars a year. Many people lack the educational background to discern a good study from a poor one. Many believe that if it's in print, it must be true.

A Brief Introduction to the Professional Association

The Academy of Nutrition and Dietetics is the oldest and most prominent professional organization for dietitians (it is discussed at length in Chapter 8). Among the most important functions of the Academy is the development of Standards of Practice and Standards of Professional Performance, outlining a dietetic practitioner's responsibilities for providing quality nutritional care. The standards provide individual practitioners with a systematic plan for implementing, evaluating, and adjusting performance in any area of practice.[10] See Chapter 7 for a discussion of the standards.

Because of the increasingly specialized nature of dietetic practice, the leadership of the Academy developed Dietetic Practice Groups (DPGs). DPGs provide a way for members of the association to network and share specialized information within their area or areas of interest and practice. Currently, the Academy of Nutrition and Dietetics supports 28 DPGs, which are described in Chapter 8 (**Figure 2–12**).

Another important function of the Academy is its recognition of excellence in practice through awards given annually by the national organization and by its affiliated state associations.[10] See Chapter 8 for a list and description of these awards.

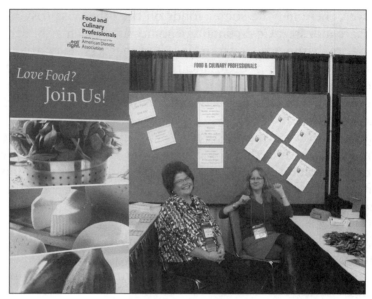

FIGURE 2–12 The Food and Culinary Professionals Dietetic Practice Group's booth at the Food and Nutrition Conference and Exposition.
Courtesy of the Academy of Nutrition and Dietetics

Summary

The horizon leans forward
Offering you space
To place new steps of change

—Excerpt from "On the Pulse of Morning," 1993
presidential inaugural poem by Maya Angelou[16]

The scope of dietetic practice is almost limitless. The creation of new, exciting positions that make use of food and nutrition education and training will continue as long as members of the profession have the imagination and determination to succeed.

"The world is happier, healthier, [and] better off because of the work you do," proclaimed Rabbi Harold S. Kushner to the dietetic professionals gathered at a recent dietetic association national conference.[17] The work of dietetics is considered a profession because it requires a specialized body of knowledge; because members render specialized services to society; because their obligations to serve override personal considerations; and because members consider competence, honor, continuing education, research, and sharing of knowledge for the common good to be necessary.

Dietetic practice encompasses nutrition therapy, the food industry, health promotion/disease prevention, foodservice systems, entrepreneurship, and education. Drawing on their training and knowledge in the fields of science, leadership, technology, research, and management, dietetic professionals communicate and collaborate to provide food and nutrition services for individuals, groups, and communities.

Dietetic practitioners work in private practice or in a hospital, with patients referred by physicians for help in implementing necessary nutritional modifications. Dietetic practitioners serve as consultants in corporate wellness programs, weight-loss programs, and eating disorder clinics. Professional athletes and athletic teams often have full-time dietitians on their training staff.

Dietetic practitioners are also involved in scientific research and education. Increasing numbers of dietitians have careers in sales, marketing, and public relations for the food industry, pharmaceutical and computer companies, and equipment manufacturers. They are involved in many areas of community work, especially with pregnant women, women with infants and young children, and the elderly.

Dietetic practitioners are particularly qualified to manage foodservice operations in hospitals, nursing homes, colleges and universities, public schools, commercial restaurants, correctional facilities, catering operations, airline commissaries, and community programs. Interest is growing in combining nutrition credentials with other degrees, such as those in business, law, nursing, physical fitness, and the culinary arts.

The Academy of Nutrition and Dietetics has developed DPGs to enable members to network and increase their knowledge within their particular area of practice. The Academy also offers annual awards for excellence in specific areas of practice and develops and promotes standards of practice that outline a dietetic practitioner's responsibilities for providing quality nutritional care.

Societal needs are best served by having a population that is adequately nourished. Dietetics serves people by offering correct and current information so that individuals can make their own choices. The education, training, and knowledge of dietitians make them uniquely qualified to help individuals and society meet their nutritional needs.

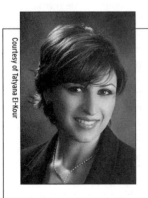
Courtesy of Tatyana El-Kour

Profile of a Professional
Tatyana El-Kour, MS, RD
National Program Officer for Healthy Lifestyles Promotion and Disease Prevention
World Health Organization, Amman, Jordan
Education:
BS in Nutrition and Food Technology, University of Jordan, Amman, Jordan
BS in Dietetics, Kansas State University, Manhattan, Kansas
Combined MS and dietetic internship, Tufts University/ Frances Stern Nutrition Center, Tufts Medical Center, Boston, Massachusetts

How did you first hear about dietetics and decide to become a Registered Dietitian?
While I was working at Novartis Consumer Health Corporation as a Nutrition Line Specialist at the Office of the Near East, I met a few registered dietitians during my meetings. They inspired me to obtain my dietetics registration in the United States.

What was your route to registration?

I started my second BS degree from Kansas State University in their online distance dietetics program. I then came to the United States to finish up my degree on the K-State campus. My combined internship program emphasized medical nutrition therapy with an elective in nutrition policy, and my master's degree was in nutrition sciences.

What are some examples of your professional involvement?

My professional involvement continues to be very important to me. While a student, I was president of the Massachusetts Student Dietetic Association, and since my student days I have been a member of the Academy of Nutrition and Dietetics and active in public policy positions. I have been president of the American Overseas Dietetic Association and an active member of dietetic practice groups within the Academy. I've served as an abstract reviewer for the Academy's national Food and Nutrition Conference and Exhibition for 3 years. In my position with WHO, I have been an appointed member on three national taskforce committees (Tobacco Control, Non-Communicable Diseases, and Nutrition in Complex Emergencies); an appointed abstract reviewer for the Tobacco Control Track for the 2010 World Cancer Congress, International Union Against Cancer, and an appointed member, International Committee, Association for Treatment of Tobacco Use and Dependence.

What honors or awards have you received?

Young Professional of the Year Award, College of Human Ecology, Kansas State University

Recognized Young Dietitian of the Year Award for Massachusetts

Friedman School of Nutrition Science and Policy Graduation Class Valedictorian

Rebecca Roubenoff Award for Excellence in Clinical Nutrition and Dietetics, Tufts Medical Center

Outstanding Dietetic Intern Award, Academy of Nutrition and Dietetics

First International Nutritionist/Dietitian Award, Academy of Nutrition and Dietetics Foundation

Briefly describe your career path in dietetics. What are you doing now?

In 1999 and immediately following my graduation from the University of Jordan, I joined Jordan Drugstore Company, a leading drugstore company in Jordan, as a medical representative for 1 year. I was mainly responsible for marketing and sales of certain drugs and nutritional supplements. A year later, I joined Novartis Consumer Health Corporation as a Nutrition Line Specialist and took over the management of medical nutrition products, infant nutrition, and functional foods in five markets of the Near East. During my second year of work at Novartis, I joined K-State's distance education dietetics program, eventually moving to the United States to complete my didactic requirements and further my graduate studies while becoming an RD.

Since my graduation from Tufts University in 2005, I have been working with WHO, Jordan Country Office, in the capacity of a temporary nutrition advisor. In the meantime, I ran an ad hoc private practice offering consultation on specific medical nutrition therapy issues designed to treat critical care, chronic, metabolic and rare conditions and disorders, including tube-feeding recommendations and behavior change. In 2008, I became a national program officer for health promotion and disease prevention programs. Being in a small country office, I work to integrate and implement nutrition programs within the realm of noncommunicable diseases, maternal and child health, and school health programs. In 2009, I obtained a formal certification in Tobacco Treatment Specialty. I also obtained board certification in nutrition support to assist me in integrating nutrition support within WHO's patient safety initiatives.

In addition to nutrition, I have been strongly involved in tobacco-control activities as well, but also handled various projects relating to violence, injuries, and disabilities. I have contributed to the writing of numerous national and international proposals, and currently conduct various projects relating to nutrition and wellness for private- and public-sector employees in Jordan. I am also spearheading a community nutrition project on preservation of traditional foods while incorporating cost-effective and nutrient-dense recipe amendments to help people eat healthfully.

What excites you about dietetics and the future of our profession?
Wherever we are—in clinics, hospitals, communities, outpatient or long-term care settings, in sports, education, government, research, or the restaurant and food industry—our work is tremendously important to the health and well-being of people.

Why/how is teamwork important to you in your position? How have you been involved in team projects?
Teamwork is crucial to develop and successfully implement a number of health promotion programs, such as healthy lifestyle programs on nutrition, tobacco control, physical activity, violence, and road safety. These programs were a major undertaking, requiring a great deal of thought and effort while maintaining a spirit of effective communication. Oftentimes in my position—as I serve as WHO liaison to many WHO collaborative programs in the Ministry of Health, other UN agencies, and NGOs—a great amount of teamwork is required. I also coordinate projects involving numerous stakeholders, and my ability to work collaboratively while guiding the projects quickly and effectively was critical.

What words of wisdom do you have for future dietetics professionals?
Do not be afraid to try new things and adventures. As Kobi Yamada said, "Sometimes you just have to take the leap and build your wings on the way down."

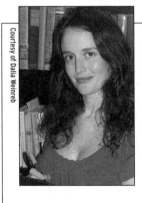

Courtesy of Dalia Weinreb

Profile of a Professional

Dalia Weinreb, RD
Registered Dietitian in private practice, Austin, Texas
Education:
BS in Environmental Biogeoscience, from the University of Leeds, United Kingdom
Met Academy academic requirements, Hunter College, New York, New York
Dietetic Internship, New York Presbyterian Hospital, New York, New York

How did you first hear about dietetics and decide to become a registered dietitian?
I discovered the power of nutrition when I figured out how to treat a digestive problem I had by modifying my diet. After seeing firsthand the fundamental role nutrition plays in promoting health, I decided that I wanted to devote my life to helping people use nutrition as "preventative medicine." Once I researched how to become qualified, I realized that the most reliable nutrition qualification was to become a registered dietitian.

Briefly describe your career path in dietetics. What are you doing now?
My aim was always to go into private practice. I most enjoy being my own boss, devising my own techniques, and seeing results on a one-to-one level. As soon as I qualified, I opened a private practice in coordination with other health professionals. I now work in a mind–body therapeutic center as a nutritionist, along with psychotherapists and psychologists. I also work independently as a nutritionist and run a weight-loss support group for people who have a stubborn overweight problem. I am currently working on starting a type 2 diabetes support group also.

What excites you about dietetics and the future of our profession?
I am so very excited about the emergence of nutrigenomics. I love to individualize the plans I devise for my clients to suit their needs, and knowledge of a person's genome will enhance this technique to an incredible level. I am also very excited about the rebirth of traditional agriculture (organic foods), eating seasonally and locally, and getting back in touch with the food chain. It is wonderful to see that best-seller lists such as those found in *The New York Times* contain books written for the layman that concern eating healthily for the body and the land. I am excited to see the population step away from their attraction to fad diets and return to wholesome eating. Dietetics is a rapidly expanding field, and I am delighted to be a part of it.

Why/how is teamwork important to you in your position? How have you been involved in team projects?
Teamwork is very important to me, even though most of my work is done as an individual professional. I work in a multidisciplinary team where I am the sole nutritionist, and I love to bring nutrition knowledge to my coworkers. For example, I enjoy showing psychotherapists the power that healthy eating and exercise have in helping heal depression in susceptible individuals. Hand in hand, we all make a great difference in our clients' lives.

What words of wisdom do you have for future dietetics professionals?
Follow your instinct. There is a vast world, full of opportunity, for dietetics professionals. Sometimes when you're learning a particular course required in your academic program, you may feel that it's not for you. Don't be disheartened. In order to become an RD, you need to learn a vast range of subjects, from management to medical nutrition therapy. Learn as much as you can, while listening to what your instinct says interests you the most. Try and choose an internship that supports your interests, and once you have your RD, follow your passion. You will only succeed and give the best help to people if you love what you do!

Suggested Activities

1. Dietetic Practice Groups (DGPs) are a good way to network with professionals who work in specific areas of dietetics. Visit www.eatright .org or refer to Chapter 8 of this book for a complete listing of the 28 DPGs. Choose one of the DPGs you might be interested in joining later in your career. If possible, attend one of the meetings of this practice group at a national meeting of the Academy of Nutrition and Dietetics or at a regional meeting. Or, interview a member of the practice group to find out what the practice group does to benefit the profession and its individual members.

2. Add to the list of specialty areas of dietetic practice discussed in the chapter either by listing positions you know exist or by developing areas of practice or positions you would be interested in personally. Be creative!

3. Visit www.eatright.org to verify the accuracy of information in this chapter. Has anything changed since this chapter was written?

4. Interested in private practice? Two-thirds of Americans either run their own business or dream of being their own boss. If you are interested in starting your own private practice, visit www.morebusiness.com, click "Tips and Tools" on the main menu, then click "6 Vital Entrepreneur

Skills for a Successful Small Business." Evaluate your own personal characteristics. Do they match those considered to be important for entrepreneurial success? Explain. Are you more or less interested in private practice after completing this exercise? Explain. If your answer was "more interested," then you may want to take a look at www.inc.com and click "Start-Up." This site offers many practical tips and good advice for starting your own business.

5. Interested in a career in foodservice management? Visit the website www.foodservice.com and click "Search Jobs." Which of them might be of interest to you in the future, or now? View a couple of the jobs to see what information is available online about these positions.

6. The salary differences for the various areas of the country may be related to the cost-of-living index in these areas. If you are unsure of what the cost-of-living index is, do an Internet search to find the cost-of-living index and its relationship to the consumer price index. Look up the cities and states listed in this chapter as having the highest and lowest salaries and compare them with the cost-of-living indexes listed for these cities on the Internet.

7. Some of the statistics and facts contained in this chapter may change as a result of economic conditions and other mitigating factors. Go to the Bureau of Labor Statistics website at www.bls.gov and research the latest information from the government on the job outlook for positions in which you have an interest. How does the information differ from that contained in the chapter?

8. Read the Code of Ethics in Chapter 7. As a future dietetic professional, what are some of the ways you could demonstrate that you have met the criteria for Standard 3 (The dietetics practitioner considers the health, safety, and welfare of the public at all times.)? Be sure that you have listed outcomes and/or goals that are specific and measurable.

9. What kinds of positions are available right now? Two companies started by dietitians provide job listings and placement services. Visit their websites at www.jobsindietetics.com and www.nutritionjobs.com. What positions are currently available? What area of dietetics are they in? Where are they located? What kinds of salaries are being offered?

10. What, in your opinion, should the dietetics profession do to address some of the issues facing practitioners today?

Selected Websites

- www.bls.gov—U.S. Department of Labor Bureau of Labor Statistics offers information on jobs and salaries across the United States.
- www.computrition.com—Computrition Foodservice Software Solutions sells computer software for the healthcare and hospitality industries.
- www.eatright.org—The Academy of Nutrition and Dietetics is the world's largest organization of food and nutrition professionals.

- www.helmpublishing.com—Helm Publishing provides continuing education for dietitians and nurses.
- www.inc.com—Inc. offers small business resources for the entrepreneur.
- www.jobsindietetics.com—Features jobs in dietetics and career services for professionals in dietetics, nutrition, and foodservice.
- www.morebusiness.com—Offers advice for entrepreneurs.
- www.nutritionjobs.com—Features career services for professionals in dietetics, nutrition, and foodservice.
- www.sfm-online.org—Society of Foodservice Management is a professional organization for those working in the foodservice industry.

Suggested Readings

Crosby O, Moncarz R. The 2004–14 job outlook for college graduates. *Occupational Outlook Quarterly*. Available at: http://www.bls.gov/opub/ooq/2006/fall/art03.pdf. Accessed January 12, 2010.

Cullen LT. Now hiring! *Time* 2003;162(21):49–53.

Harnack L, French S. Fattening up on fast food. *J Am Diet Assoc*. 2003;103(10):1296–1297.

King K. *Helm Publishing: Books and Continuing Education for RDs, DTRs & RNs*. Lake Dallas, TX: Helm Publishing; Winter–Spring 2004.

Krieger E, Mantel C, Morreale S. Business and communications: career opportunities for dietitians. Presentation at ADA Food and Nutrition Conference & Expo. San Antonio, TX: October 2003.

Los Angeles Times. Menu of jobs available in the restaurant industry. *Careerbuilder*. December 7, 2003. www.careerbuilder.com

Los Angeles Times. Restaurant workers step up to the plate: jobs covering a range of duties available in changing industry. *Careerbuilder*. December 7, 2003. www.careerbuilder.com

McCluskey KW. Customer service in health care—dietetics professionals can take the lead. *J Am Diet Assoc*. 2003;103(10):1282.

Occupational Outlook Handbook, 2010–11. U.S. Bureau of Labor Statistics website. www.bls.gov/ooh. Accessed February 23, 2013.

O'Sullivan Maillet J. Dietetics in 2017: what does the future hold? *J Am Diet Assoc*. 2002; 10:1404–1407.

Schofield M. Professional issues delegate's column: Future dimensions. *Clin Nutr Manage*. 2003;22:14.

Smith Edge M. President's page: leading the future of dietetics. *J Am Diet Assoc*. 2003; 103:420.

Smith Edge M. President's page: promote the profession and market our services: an ADA team effort. *J Am Diet Assoc*. 2003;103(10):1276.

Spotlight on nutrition innovators: DTRs pioneer new arenas. *J Am Diet Assoc*. 2003;103(10):1279–1280.

Tactical Workgroup of the ADA House of Delegates. Performance, proficiency, and value of dietetics professional: an update. *J Am Diet Assoc*. 2003;103(10):1376–1379.

References

1. *Collins English Dictionary*, 6th ed. New York: HarperCollins; 2003.
2. *Mosby's Medical Dictionary*, 8th ed. Philadelphia: Elsevier; 2009.
3. American Dietetic Association. *2009 Compensation and Benefits Survey of the American Dietetic Association*. Chicago: The American Dietetic Association; 2010.

4. Brandeis LD. *Business—A profession*. University of Louisville, Louis D. Brandeis School of Law website. http://www.law.louisville.edu/library/collections/brandeis/node/202. Accessed April 26, 2010.

5. The American Dietetic Association Committee on Goals of Education for Dietetics. Goals of the lifetime education of the dietitian. *J Am Diet Assoc*. 1969;54:91–93.

6. Galbraith A. Excellence defined. *J Am Diet Assoc*. 1975;67:211.

7. Health professionals. Academy of Nutrition and Dietetics website. http://www.eatright .org/HealthProfessionals/. Accessed February 18, 2010.

8. Academy of Nutrition and Dietetics website. http://www.eatright.org/scope/. Accessed February 22, 2013. Used with permission of the Academy of Nutrition & Dietetics, 2013. Note: The Definition of Terms is a cumulative anthology of definitions developed by the Academy of Nutrition and Dietetics (Academy). The definitions are broad based, have implications for use across the nutrition and dietetics profession, and are consistent with the regulatory and legal needs of the profession. The terms are a resource for registered dietitians, dietetic technicians, registered, and other food and nutrition practitioners as applicable. As a reference document, the definitions serve as standardized language and standardized application in various practice settings.

9. American Dietetic Association. Hornick BA, ed. *Job Descriptions: Models for the Dietetics Profession*. Chicago: The American Dietetic Association; 2003.

10. Academy of Nutrition and Dietetics website. http://www.eatright.org. Accessed January 22, 2010.

11. Paddock C. Obesity healthcare costs US 147 billion dollars a year, new study. *Medical News Today*. Available at: http://www.medicalnewstoday.com/articles/158948.php. Accessed January 20, 2010.

12. Thottam J. Health kick. *Time* 2003;16221:54–57.

13. Crosby O, Moncarz R. The 2004–2014 job outlook for college graduates. *Occupational Outlook Quarterly* Online. Available at: http://www.bls.gov/opub/ooq/2006/fall/art03 .pdf. Accessed January 12, 2010.

14. Bureau of Labor Statistics. The 2004–2014 job outlook in brief. *Occupational Outlook Quarterly* Online. Available at: http:www.bls.gov/ooh. Accessed February 23, 2013.

15. Bureau of Labor Statistics. The 2006–2016 job outlook in brief. *Occupational Outlook Quarterly* Online. Available at: http://www.bls.gov/opub/ooq/2008/spring/art01.pdf. Accessed January 12, 2010.

16. Angelou M. *On the Pulse of Morning*. New York: Random House; 1993.

17. American Dietetic Association. *Set Your Sights: Your Future in Dietetics*. Chicago: The American Dietetic Association; 1991.

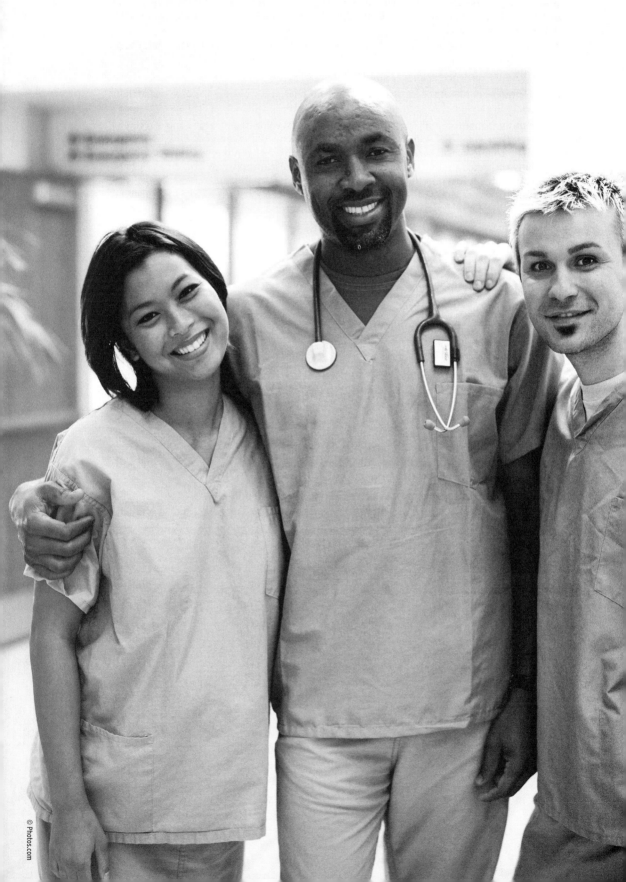

Joining Together: The Team Approach

Have you ever heard someone say, "I prefer to work alone"? Well, they might as well forget it. Work in the twenty-first century will be done in groups and teams, specifically:

> In all healthcare settings more work is being done by versatile and flexible multidisciplinary teams that plan, implement, and review cases. Members are valued for their ability to help the team with a "flexible eye" in making judgments and pitching in to do what needs to be done. The most valued members are those with a global view of health and proficiency in a greater number of competencies. Teams reduce costs by using fewer employees, using them synergistically, and pushing care toward lower-paid practitioners.[1]

Because of this, it is now essential that dietetics professionals be multi-skilled, cross-trained, and effective team players.

Long gone are the days of the family doctor acting alone to treat disease. Today, a career in health care is no longer limited to being either a doctor or nurse. The U.S. healthcare system is one of the most sophisticated and complex in the world. The increase in the number of older adults, shortages in the healthcare workforce, the emergence of specialized treatments that require complex technology, a new focus on preventive health care, and a better understanding of the cost benefits of a healthy workforce all create very positive prospects for anyone entering a healthcare career and serving on successful healthcare teams.

The explosion of scientific knowledge has led to a corresponding increase in the number of healthcare professions that require specialized knowledge and skills. The term *allied health* is used to describe a cluster of roles in the healthcare system that assist, facilitate, and complement the work of physicians, nurses, and pharmacists. The American Society of Allied Health Professions lists more than 100 different health service careers.[2] For example, the data acquired by laboratory technicians plays a crucial role in the detection, diagnosis, and treatment of disease. The medical records administrator collects, analyzes, and manages information that steers the healthcare industry. The rehabilitation process for a patient often requires the combined efforts of physical therapists, medical social workers, occupational therapists, speech therapists, and dietitians. The hospital pharmacist works with nurses, doctors, and dietitians to provide quality patient care. These specialty areas free highly skilled medical practitioners—physicians, nurses, and pharmacists—to perform the tasks they alone are qualified to do.

In one report, a healthcare team was composed of geriatric, infectious disease, heart, and cancer physician specialists; nurses at various levels of specialization and care; physical, occupational, speech, and respiratory therapists; a dietitian; a chaplain; and a social worker. The tightly coordinated diagnosis and care by this 14-member team saved the patient's life. At the same time, each of the members of this team served on other teams with different memberships to provide care and rehabilitation to other patients. Their ability to work together on teams was the key to their success.[3]

The team approach has been used successfully in the treatment of adolescents with eating disorders. One pediatric eating disorders team might include a physician who specializes in treating the malnutrition of eating disorders and who is trained in adolescent medicine, a registered dietitian trained in adolescent medicine, a nurse, a mental health professional such as a psychiatrist or psychologist, a licensed social worker, a licensed counselor, and an advanced practice nurse.[4]

The History of the Healthcare Team Concept

The concept of the healthcare team emerged after World War II, a period of increased social awareness and higher healthcare expectations. Disabled veterans returning from the war required more than traditional medical treatment for their physical disabilities. They also needed assistance in returning to the community as socially and economically useful citizens. This led to a trend toward sharing responsibilities with other professionals that had formerly been the sole purview of the physician and/or nurse. This trend has had a major impact on the quality, costs, organization, and delivery of health care.

What Makes a Group a Team?

A **group** may be very simply defined as two or more individuals interacting with each other in such a manner that each person influences and is influenced by each other person. A group is not a team. A **team** is a small number of people with complementary skills who are committed to a common purpose, performance goals, and approach for which they hold themselves mutually accountable.[5] Two important characteristics distinguish a team from a group: (1) a team produces specific results for which the team is *collectively* responsible, and (2) a team possesses *super-consciousness* of being a team, an awareness of needing each other.[6]

Teamwork

Teamwork is the close, cooperative effort of several people to use their special skills and knowledge to meet the needs of the client/patient more efficiently, completely, competently, and considerately than would be possible by individual, independent action. An important, but often forgotten, member of the team is the client/patient.

Educating and including the client/patient in the team communication process are critically important. Because the ultimate responsibility for client/patient care rests with the physician, it is the physician who assumes the leadership role on most healthcare teams. Other members of the team vary, depending on the needs of the client/patient. A chart of possible members of a healthcare team for a patient with lung cancer is shown in **Figure 3–1**.

To function effectively, the members of healthcare teams must be able to differentiate between roles that are unique to each discipline and roles that are shared. Team members function independently when they have unique competencies, knowledge, and experiences. **Delegated functioning** occurs when the team has varying levels and types of training.

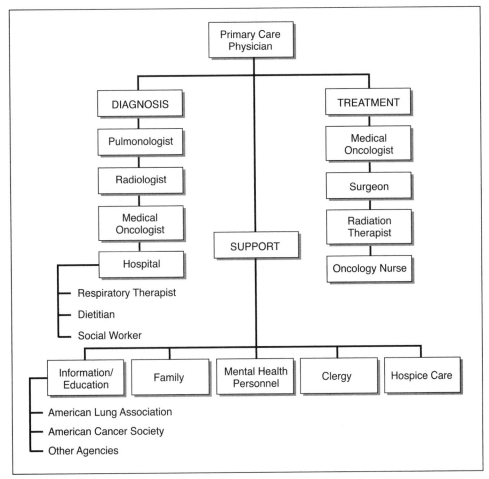

FIGURE 3–1 An organization chart showing possible members of a healthcare team for a patient with lung cancer.

Collaborative functioning is used when an overlap in competencies allows for a common base for judgment and decision making.

A clinical dietitian doing a patient discharge diet instruction is functioning independently. A delegated function for this same dietitian would be the implementation of a physician-prescribed diet order. An example of a collaborative, multidisciplinary approach would be the implementation of a weight-control program involving a physician, a dietitian, an exercise physiologist, a laboratory technician, and a psychologist. Diseases that have systemic effects are natural candidates for the collaborative, multidisciplinary team approach. For example, care for patients with diabetes often involves a primary care physician, an endocrinologist, a dietitian, a nurse/nurse practitioner, an ophthalmologist, a podiatrist, a health educator, and others.

Fundamentals of Team Dynamics

Unfortunately, in today's work environment team members' teamwork skills often lag far behind their technical skills. An understanding of the fundamentals of team dynamics, team development, team planning, team communication, and leadership sharing is an important adjunct to a professional's technical knowledge.

A team was previously defined in this chapter as "a small number of people with complementary skills who are committed to a common purpose, performance goals, and approach for which they hold themselves mutually accountable." Careful analysis of this definition reveals four important dimensions (**Figure 3–2**). First, a team should comprise a small number of people. Second, the team members must have complementary skills.

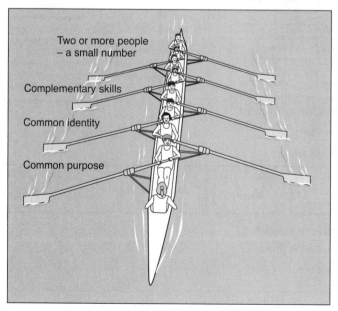

FIGURE 3–2 What does it take to make a team?

Third, there must be general consensus on why the team exists. Finally, the team members hold themselves mutually accountable for the work and results of the team's efforts.

Types of Teams

People are on groups and teams for many different reasons. Sometimes team membership is an end in itself. Many leisure activities lend themselves to team activities for the purpose of socializing. Cycling teams and basketball teams are just two examples of informal teams that satisfy social needs for working adults. Thus, an *informal team* can be defined as a team whose principal reason for existence is to provide friendship. People join such teams to have a sense of belonging, of acceptance, of recognition, and of being liked by others. Such teams usually do not have an officially appointed leader, although informal leadership often develops by popular acclaim. Informal teams usually develop spontaneously and may over time evolve into formal teams.[7]

Formal teams are created to achieve performance goals that, in turn, contribute to the success of the larger organization. Formal teams are more rationally structured and less fluid than informal ones. Rather than choosing to join, as in the case of informal teams, individuals are usually assigned to formal work teams because of their expertise and the needs of the team. One person is usually granted formal leadership responsibility.[7]

However, research has shown that in every high-performance team, leadership is shared.[5] This means that even though there is a designated leadership position, each member of the team shares responsibility for facilitating the team's work (**Figure 3–3**).

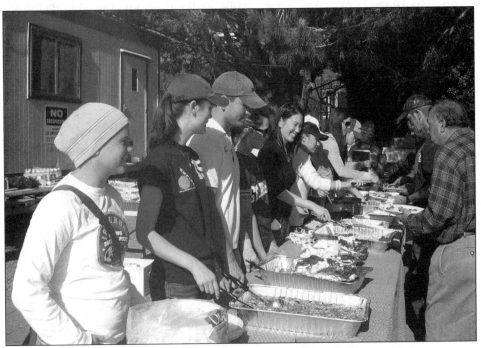

FIGURE 3–3 Nutrition students serving a lunch they prepared for a local labor exchange.
Courtesy of Lisa Ching, RD

Attraction to Teams, Roles, and Norms

Commitment to a team is said to hinge on two factors: attractiveness ("the outside looking in" view) and cohesiveness ("the inside looking out" view), or the tendency of the group to stick together and resist outside influences. A relatively small team of members who share similar traits with a high degree of interaction and cooperative relationships and who have a superior public image and enjoy prestige and status are the most likely to be attractive and cohesive. Unpleasant experiences and disagreements within the team, unreasonable demands made on team members, an unfavorable public image, and competition for membership and time all have a negative impact on attractiveness and cohesiveness.[8]

Also important to the functioning of a team is the concept of role. A **role** is defined as a socially determined prescription for behavior in a specific position. Every employee has one or more organizational roles to play. One key to organizational and team success is for everyone to play his or her role effectively and efficiently. Roles usually focus on a specific position, whereas norms are broader in scope.[9] **Norms** are general standards of conduct that help individuals judge what is right or wrong or good or bad; as such, they influence behavior enormously (**Figure 3–4**).[10]

Every team, whether informal or formal, develops its own set of norms that are enforced for the following reasons:

1. To ensure survival of the team

2. To simplify or clarify role expectations

3. To help team members avoid embarrassing situations and protect self-images

4. To express key team values and enhance the team's unique identification[11]

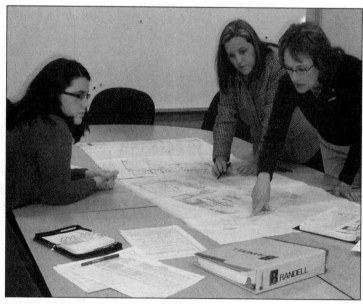

Figure 3–4 A facility design team, including a dietitian, collaborating on a project.
Courtesy of Christine Guyott, RD

Team Development

A group does not become a team overnight. The first few meetings of a new team may be fraught with a sense of uneasiness; lack of trust; uncertainty about roles, objectives, and leadership; and even defensive behavior and differences of opinion. Management experts have identified six stages of team development: orientation, conflict and challenge, cohesion, delusion, disillusion, and acceptance. During the first three stages, attempts are made to overcome uncertainty with regard to power and authority. Once this obstacle has been cleared, stages 4 through 6 address the uncertainty over interpersonal relationships. Teams that reach stage 6 are highly effective and efficient mature teams.[12]

The following are some important characteristics of mature teams:

1. Members are aware of their own and each other's assets and liabilities with regard to the team's task.

2. Individual differences are accepted without being labeled as good or bad.

3. The team has developed authority and interpersonal relationships that are recognized and accepted by the members.

4. Team decisions are made through rational discussion. Minority opinions and dissension are recognized and encouraged. Attempts are not made to force decisions or create a false unanimity.

5. Conflict is over substantive team issues such as team goals and the effectiveness and efficiency of various means for achieving those goals. Conflict over emotional issues regarding team structure, processes, or interpersonal relationships is at a minimum.

6. Members are aware of the team's processes and their own roles in them.[12]

Communicating for Team Success

Communication is the glue that binds the behavior among the members of the team. Communication can be defined as the constant development of understanding among people. Effective communication means that there is successful transfer of information, meaning, and understanding from a sender to a receiver. It is not necessary to have agreement, but there must be mutual understanding for the exchange to be considered successful.[13]

Types of Communication

Oral communication is the most common form of team communication and is generally superior to other forms of communication. Oral communication takes less time and is more effective in achieving understanding. Face-to-face communication has the advantage of also providing information through body language, personal mannerisms, and facial expressions.

Other types of communication include written communication, visual aids, gestures, and actions. Visual aids, such as pictures, charts, cartoons, symbols, and videos, can be particularly effective when used with good oral communication.

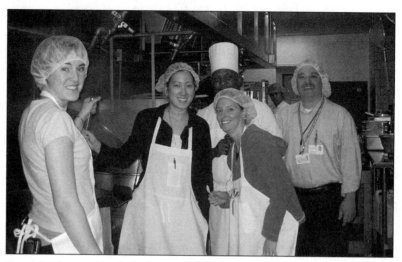

FIGURE 3–5 An executive chef, a foodservice manager, and interns team up on a meal project.
Courtesy of Jennifer Chang, RD

"Actions speak louder than words" is sage advice for any manager. Gestures, handshakes, a shrug of the shoulders, a smile, and silence all have meaning and are powerful forms of communication to team members (**Figure 3–5**).

Barriers to Good Communication

Some barriers to communication have to do with the language used, the differing backgrounds of the sender and receiver, and the circumstances in which the communication takes place. The receiver may hear what he or she expects to hear and may shut out or ignore that which is unexpected or conflicts. The receiver also has a tendency to infer what is expected even when it is not communicated. Receivers are also susceptible to information overload, which occurs when someone receives more information than he or she is able to process.

Receivers evaluate the source and interpret or accept communication in light of that evaluation. A trusted and respected team member will have more open channels of communication than a team member who does not command trust and respect.

Different people often attach various meanings to certain words. The sender or communicator not only must choose words that convey the meaning to the receiver, but also must give attention to the message transmitted by nonverbal cues. Body language and facial expression often say more than the words they accompany.

A receiver who is emotionally upset often stops listening in order to think about what he or she will say next. Noise and the environment may form a physical barrier to communication. Time and place are also important. There is a right place and a wrong place to conduct good communication, just as there is a right time and a wrong time. Time pressures on the sender form a barrier to effective communication because of hastily developed messages, use of the most expedient rather than the most effective channel, and insufficient time for feedback.

A network breakdown occurs when there is a disruption or closure of a communication channel. This can be caused by a number of factors, both intentional and unintentional. Some reasons for the network to break down are forgetfulness, jealousy, fear of negative feedback, and a desire to gain an edge over the competition.

Improving Communication

Communication is not a one-way process. One of the most important parts of effective communication is to listen to the reply, which may entail words, facial expressions, body language, and even silence. The evaluation of feedback can tell much about how the message has been received. Empathy—the ability to put yourself in the receiver's shoes in a conversation—is crucial to mutual understanding.

Face-to-face communication is advantageous because of the ability to gain immediate feedback from multiple channels, such as oral expression, facial expressions, and body language. To secure understanding, it is often effective to repeat the information using slightly different words, phrases, or approaches. Being sensitive to the receiver can improve communication. Some words or phrases have symbolic meaning to others, and these words should be avoided. Proper timing is also important. The old maxim "criticize in private, praise in public" is an example of timing. Reinforcing words with congruent actions has already been discussed as essential to effective communication. Finally, an atmosphere of openness and trust, fostered by self-disclosure, builds healthy relationships that contribute to effective communication in a team setting.[13]

Productive Communication

Teamwork requires productive communication that supports and encourages authentic, inclusive sharing and negotiation of ideas and perspectives. When this occurs, a climate develops in which members are sensitive to one another, dialogue is supported, and defensiveness is reduced through language that is **assertive, responsible, confirming**, and **appropriate**.[13]

Sensitivity means being able to understand other team members' feelings and responses and to adapt the response accordingly. People who are able to do this are flexible, assertive, and not bound by predetermined gender roles.[14]

Note that assertiveness is not aggressiveness. Aggressive communication is an attempt to control others, with a low regard for their interests or feelings. **Assertive communication** is open, with an awareness of self and concern for others. Even though assertiveness is often direct, it is also very gentle and considerate of others' opinions. Team members who are assertive focus on problems, not on people, and on openness, not on strategy or manipulation. Being assertive means taking some risks, knowing and stating your position responsibly and openly, and being sensitive to others' responses.

Responsible communication means taking responsibility for one's feelings and ideas. Some years ago it was suggested that "I statements" are a more responsible way of communicating. Starting a statement with "you" rather than "I" implies that someone else is to blame; for example, saying "You're always late" versus "I feel frustrated that you are often late." Absolute terms such as "always" and "never" should also be avoided.[15]

Confirming communication means listening to, acknowledging, and understanding the ideas and feelings of others. This is often accomplished with statements like "That's a good idea" or "Tell us more about that." Such statements are called person-centered messages, and they confirm a person's worth and role in a process. A person who uses person-centered messages is seen as more persuasive.[16] The opposite of confirmation is rejection or disconfirming, which may be communicated with silence, changing the subject, or an impersonal response.[17]

Appropriate communication means using dialogue that opens up the discussion and understanding. It means using language that fits the team members, yourself, and the team context. Appropriate communication means being clear and concrete and speaking at the listeners' knowledge level.[3]

A team that has mastered the art of productive communication should be able to say:

- We support and confirm one another so that everyone speaks and is heard.
- We respect one another's differences and adapt our communication to open up discussion.
- We take care to express our ideas responsibly and appropriately.
- We consider and refine our thinking with careful negotiation and definition of terms.[3]

What Makes a Work Team Effective?

Based on a number of studies, the determinants of team effectiveness may be grouped into three categories: people-related factors, organization-related factors, and task-related factors.

People-Related Factors

Personal work satisfaction

Mutual trust and team spirit

Good communication

Low unresolved conflict and power struggle

Low threat, fail-safe, good job security

Organization-Related Factors

Organizational stability and job security

Involved, interested, supportive management

Stable goals and priorities

Task-Related Factors

Clear objectives, directions, and plans

Proper technical direction and leadership

Autonomy and professionally challenging work

Experienced and qualified team personnel

Team involvement and work visibility

The presence of these determinants leads to effective team performance characterized by:

- Accomplishment of goals
- Adaptability to change
- High personal/team commitment
- High rating by upper management
- Generation of innovative ideas[18]

Among the people-related factors, one stands out as being key to effective teamwork and requires careful attention in today's work milieu—trust. **Trust** is the belief in the integrity, character, or ability of others. Trust is a fragile entity. Earning a person's trust is a long, slow process that can be destroyed in an instant with a careless remark. In the team process, the primary responsibility for building a climate of trust belongs to the team leader, but each member of the team shares this responsibility. There are six ways to build trust:

- **Communication.** Be open and honest, provide timely feedback, and keep people informed.
- **Support.** Be approachable and available to help, encourage, and coach.
- **Respect.** Delegate important duties and be a good listener.
- **Fairness.** Evaluate people fairly and objectively, be liberal in giving credit and praise.
- **Predictability.** Be dependable and consistent in your behavior, keep promises and deadlines.
- **Competence.** Be technically and professionally competent, be a good role model.

Although concentration on these six areas is advised for team leaders, they are equally important for team members. In addition, those who feel trusted tend to trust others in return.[7]

Members of Healthcare Teams

There are more than 100 possible members of the healthcare team![19] This section highlights a few of the professionals who may be included on the healthcare team. Members of the dietetic team form a subset of the larger healthcare team and are discussed first. Members of the dietetic team can most often be found working in the organizational healthcare setting. Dietitians, dietetic technicians, and dietary managers are the primary positions that make up the dietetic team. In recent years, healthcare issues such as labor shortages, cost containment, and quality assurance have forced the dietetic team to be better coordinated and to delegate less specialized, more routine tasks to less highly trained personnel.

Dietitians

Dietitians are highly qualified professionals who are recognized experts on food and nutrition. The educational requirements to become a dietitian are described in Chapter 5. The Academy of Nutrition and Dietetics is the primary professional association for dietitians and dietetic technicians. Dietitians work in a wide variety of settings, most of which fall into nine categories, discussed next.

Dietitians in Business. Dietitians in business work in areas such as food manufacturing, advertising, and marketing. Dietitians who work for food manufacturers or grocery chains may analyze the nutrition content for foods for labeling purposes or marketing efforts. They may also prepare literature for distribution to customers and write articles for the news media. To satisfy consumers' growing interest in nutrition, dietitians are employed by businesses to develop new products, sell and market products, and develop public relations and advertising programs. Many entrepreneurial dietitians have developed a product, product line, or service themselves and have built a company to market and sell the products or services (**Figure 3–6**).

Clinical Dietitians. Clinical dietitians provide nutritional services for patients in hospitals, nursing homes, clinics, health maintenance organizations (HMOs), doctors' offices, and other healthcare facilities. They assess patients' nutritional needs, develop and implement nutrition programs, and evaluate and report the results. They are a vital part of the healthcare team, working with doctors and other healthcare professionals to coordinate nutritional intake with other treatments, such as medications (**Figure 3–7**).

Many clinical dietitians specialize in one area of practice. Diabetes, heart disease, pediatrics, geriatrics, renal disease, the critically ill, and obesity are some of the areas in which clinical dietitians specialize. Nutritional care of the critically ill, for example, involves overseeing patients requiring tube or intravenous feedings. Clinical dietitians working with patients with diabetes teach them how to establish and adhere to a long-term nutrition program and how to monitor blood glucose levels.

In addition to assessing patients' nutrition needs and developing treatment plans, clinical dietitians have administrative and managerial duties. In a small nursing home or hospital, the clinical dietitian may run the foodservice department. In larger facilities, the clinical dietitian may supervise dietetic technicians and other support staff such as patient service supervisors, diet clerks, and clerical personnel.

Community Dietitians. Community dietitians reach out to the public to teach, monitor, and advise individuals and groups in their efforts to prevent disease and promote good health (**Figure 3–8**). They are employed by international organizations; federal, state, and local governments; food businesses;

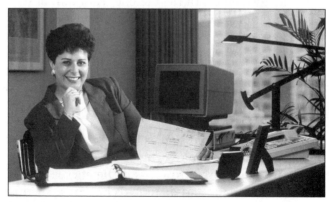

FIGURE 3–6 A dietitian who works in business.
Courtesy of the Academy of Nutrition and Dietetics

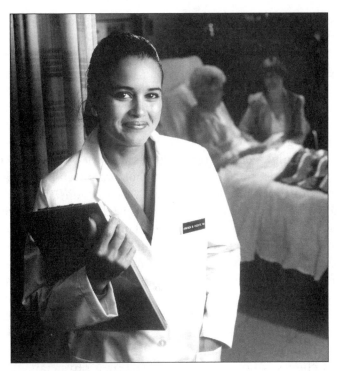

FIGURE 3–7 A clinical dietitian.
Courtesy of the Academy of Nutrition and Dietetics

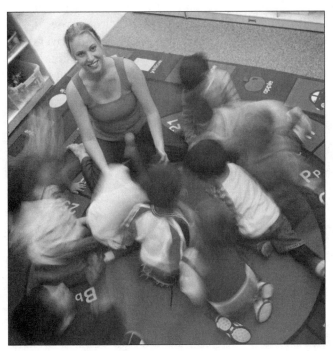

FIGURE 3–8 A community dietitian working with children.
Courtesy of the Academy of Nutrition and Dietetics

and trade associations. A variety of public, private, and volunteer organizations concerned with international health employ community nutritionists. The United Nations and the Peace Corps are just two such organizations. The U.S. Department of Agriculture, the U.S. Department of Health and Human Services, and the public health division of state and local governments employ community nutritionists to plan and carry out programs to address nutritional problems of targeted groups. The WIC (Women, Infants, and Children) program is one example. The main responsibility of community nutritionists employed by food businesses and associations is nutrition education. For example, the dairy industry has organized large-scale nutrition education programs for schoolchildren and other groups.

Community dietitians evaluate individual needs, establish nutritional care plans, and communicate the principles of good nutrition in a way that individuals and their families can understand. Teaching is a very large component of the community dietitian's job. Topics run the gamut, ranging from grocery shopping to the preparation of infant formula. They also support menu planning for those with diabetes, alcoholism, or hypertension, among many other conditions.

Consultant Dietitians. Consultant dietitians may be self-employed in their own private practice or under contract to one or more healthcare facilities. In private practice, the consultant dietitian performs nutrition screening and assessment of clients, who are often referred by a physician. Weight loss is the most common diet-related concern of clients who seek a private-practice dietitian. Consultant dietitians under contract to healthcare facilities provide expert advice on foodservice management issues such as menu planning, budgeting, cost control, portion control, sanitation, and safety. They also monitor clinical nutritional care (**Figure 3–9**).

Dietitians in Education. Dietitians in education teach the science of food and nutrition to future dietitians, dietetic technicians, dietary managers, doctors, nurses, dentists, chefs, and others. Their employers are universities, colleges, community colleges, technical schools, medical schools, dietetic internship programs, and other educational programs. Although education

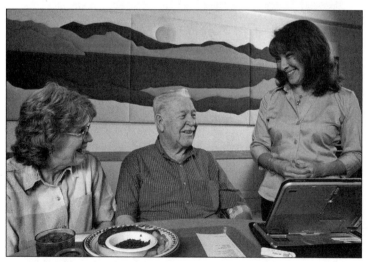

Figure 3–9 A consultant dietitian who specializes in the area of senior health.
Courtesy of the Academy of Nutrition and Dietetics

is a major component of most dietitians' job responsibilities, this category is for those who are employed by an educational institution or program, rather than an organization whose primary responsibility is health care.

Management Dietitians. Although management is a major component of most dietitians' job responsibilities, this category is for those who have the title of manager, director, or administrator. They are responsible for large-scale meal planning and preparation in such places as hospitals, nursing homes, retirement residences, company cafeterias, correctional facilities, elementary and secondary schools, food factories, colleges and universities, transportation companies, restaurants, the military, and recreational facilities.

The management dietitian supervises the planning, preparation, and service of meals; selects, trains, and directs other dietitians, foodservice supervisors, and foodservice workers; budgets for and purchases food, equipment, and supplies; enforces sanitary and safety regulations; prepares records and reports; and directs clinical services, public health nutrition, and other nutrition programs.

Dietitians who direct food and nutrition departments also decide on departmental policies and coordinate food and nutrition services with the activities of other departments. The use of computer programs to adjust recipes, prepare purchase orders, cost recipes and menus, keep inventory records, prepare financial reports, conduct nutritional analyses, and so on, has simplified many of the routine functions of management dietetics.

Research Dietitians. Research dietitians work for government agencies, food or pharmaceutical companies, academic medical centers, or educational institutions. Using the scientific method and analytical techniques, they conduct studies that range from pure to applied science. Oftentimes the research is conducted collaboratively with physicians, exercise physiologists, chemists, food technologists, and researchers from other disciplines. Research dietitians may explore the way the body uses a particular food or the interaction of drugs and diet. They may investigate the nutritional needs of individuals with different diseases or ways to reduce the risk of disease. Research in the management arena may involve the effectiveness of various foodservice systems or the efficiency of different types of foodservice equipment.

Dietetic Technicians. Dietetic technicians complete a 2-year associate degree in an Academy of Nutrition and Dietetics–approved dietetic technician program that combines both classroom and supervised practice experiences. They are then eligible to take the registration examination for dietetic technicians. Individuals who pass the exam may then use the initials DTR, for Dietetic Technician, Registered, after their name.

Dietetic technicians work in a wide variety of settings and assume an even wider variety of responsibilities. Dietetic technicians are found in hospitals, public health nutrition programs, long-term care facilities, child nutrition and school lunch programs, nutrition programs for the elderly, and foodservice management. Screening patients to identify nutritional problems, modifying menus, providing patient education and counseling to individuals and groups, developing menus and recipes, supervising foodservice personnel, purchasing food, conducting inventory, and maintaining computer systems are the most commonly performed functions of a dietetic technician.

Dietary Managers. Dietary managers are members of the Association of Nutrition & Foodservice Professionals (ANFP), formerly the Dietary Managers Association (DMA). Although no legal relationship exists between the Academy of Nutrition and Dietetics and the Association of Nutrition & Foodservice Professionals, a very close working relationship has always existed. Dietary managers have been trained in foodservice operations and usually supervise and manage dietetic service in long-term care facilities, hospitals, schools, the military, correctional institutions, and other noncommercial foodservice operations.

Other Members of the Healthcare Team

A few of the more than 100 members of the healthcare team are highlighted in this section.

PHYSICIANS   Required training for physicians includes a 4-year postgraduate medical degree (either an MD or a DO). Medical schools in the United States have specific undergraduate entrance requirements, including coursework in mathematics, the sciences, and the humanities. Entrance to medical school is very competitive and is based on undergraduate grade-point average, the results of a standardized medical school entrance exam, letters of recommendation, and community service, volunteer, or research experience.

Medical school includes 2 years of basic medical science followed by 2 years of clinical training. The clinical training concentrates heavily on the daily care of hospitalized patients. During these 2 years, medical students begin to explore areas of specialization in medicine. After graduation from medical school, doctors are required to complete a residency in a specialty, which lasts 3 to 5 years. A fellowship may follow the residency program if a doctor wants to train in a subspecialty area. For example, a residency in pediatrics could be followed by a fellowship in neonatology (care of newborns, including premature infants), pediatric cardiology (the heart and circulatory system), pediatric neurology (the brain and nervous system), pediatric hematology (the blood), pediatric oncology (cancer and tumors), pediatric gastroenterology (the digestive system), or pediatric nephrology (the kidneys).

- **Cardiology.** Cardiologists diagnose and treat cardiovascular defects and diseases. They are concerned with the structure and function of the heart and blood vessels and with the circulation of blood throughout the body.
- **Emergency medicine.** An emergency physician focuses on the immediate decision making and action necessary to prevent death or any further disability in the emergency room. The emergency physician provides immediate recognition, evaluation, care, stabilization, and disposition of patients in response to acute illness and injury.
- **Endocrinology.** An endocrinologist diagnoses and treats diseases of the hormone-producing glandular system—including the pituitary, thyroid, parathyroid, and adrenal glands and the gonads—and the insulin-producing cells of the pancreas. Endocrinologists also treat patients with metabolic disorders.

- **Family practice.** A family physician is concerned with the total health of the individual and the family and is trained to diagnose and treat a wide variety of ailments in patients of all ages. The family physician's broad training includes internal medicine, pediatrics, obstetrics and gynecology, psychiatry, and geriatrics. Special emphasis is placed on prevention and the primary care of entire families.
- **Internal medicine.** An internist provides long-term comprehensive care in the office and the hospital, managing both common and complex illnesses of all ages. Internists are trained in diagnosis and treatment of cancer, infections, and diseases affecting the heart, blood, kidneys, joints, and digestive, respiratory, and vascular systems. They are also trained in the essentials of primary care internal medicine, which includes an understanding of disease prevention, wellness, substance abuse, mental health, and the effective treatment of common problems of the eyes, ears, skin, nervous system, and reproductive organs.
- **Neurology.** An internal medicine specialty, neurology deals with disorders of the human brain, spinal cord, peripheral nerves, and muscles. Neurologists care for patients with a myriad of disorders such as pain, weakness in the arms or legs, or memory loss.
- **Obstetrics/gynecology.** An obstetrician/gynecologist has special knowledge, skills, and professional capability in the medical and surgical care of the female reproductive system and associated disorders.
- **Oncology.** An oncologist is concerned with neoplastic growth (abnormal new growth of cells and tissues), including the cause and the pattern of the abnormality.
- **Ophthalmology.** An ophthalmologist deals with the structure, function, and diseases of the eye, including medical and surgical treatment of its defects and diseases.
- **Osteopathy.** Osteopathy is a system of medical practice based on a theory that diseases are due chiefly to loss of structural integrity that can be restored by manipulation of the affected parts, supplemented by therapeutic measures (e.g., medicine, physical therapy, or surgery). During medical school, osteopathic physicians (DOs), receive extra training in the musculoskeletal system (the body's interconnected system of nerves, muscles, and bones that make up about two-thirds of the body mass). DOs are trained to be primary care physicians with a focus on preventive health care. They practice a "whole-person" approach to medicine; rather than treating specific symptoms or illnesses, they assess the overall health of the person, including home and work environments.
- **Pathology.** Pathologists provide and interpret laboratory information to help solve diagnostic problems and monitor the effects of therapy for other medical specialists.
- **Pediatrics.** Pediatricians provide preventive health maintenance for healthy children and medical care for those who are ill. Pediatricians diagnose and treat infections, injuries, genetic defects, malignancies, and many types of organic disease and dysfunction.
- **Psychiatry.** Psychiatrists specialize in the prevention, diagnosis, and treatment of mental, addictive, and emotional disorders such as

schizophrenia and other psychotic, mood, anxiety, substance-related, sexual and gender identity, and adjustment disorders.

- **Surgery.** Surgeons deal with problems by using operative procedures. The problems may be mechanical or structural (e.g., hernias, fractures, ulcers), biological (e.g., ulcers), or metabolic (e.g., an islet cell tumor of the pancreas, which causes the pancreas to secrete too much insulin). Surgical subspecialties include gastrointestinal (digestive tract), plastic surgery, vascular (blood vessels), cardiothoracic (heart and chest), pediatric (infants and children), endocrine (glands), orthopedic (bones and nervous system), otolaryngology (ear, nose, and throat), gynecology (female organs), hand, trauma and burn, oncology (cancer), and transplantation (transplanted organs).

NURSES   Registered nurses (RNs) are active in the prevention of illness in clinics, industry, and public health; the care of patients in emergency and intensive-care settings; and the care of patients in their own homes. There are more than 100 nursing specialties. The specialty may focus on a specific disease, organ/system, work setting, scope of practice, patient age, criticalness of patient condition, or technology.

Nurse Practitioners. Nurse practitioners are registered nurses with advanced formal education. Most have a master's degree in nursing and are certified by a national professional association. Working in collaboration with physicians and other members of the healthcare team, nurse practitioners obtain medical histories and perform physical exams; diagnose and treat common health problems; diagnose, treat, and monitor chronic diseases; order and interpret lab work and x-rays; provide family planning, prenatal care, well-baby and child care, and health maintenance care; conduct patient and family education and counseling programs; provide referrals to healthcare team members; and, in some states, prescribe medication.

Licensed Practical/Vocational Nurses. Licensed practical nurses (LPNs), or licensed vocational nurses (LVNs), as they are called in California and Texas, provide basic bedside care by taking vital signs, treating bedsores, preparing and giving injections and enemas, monitoring catheters, observing patients, collecting samples for testing, feeding patients, and recording food and fluid intake and output. They also help patients with bathing, dressing, and personal hygiene.

Certified Nursing Assistants. Certified nursing assistants (CNAs) perform various patient/resident care activities and related nursing functions necessary to provide for the personal needs and comfort of the facility residents/patients. CNA duties include serving meals, nourishments, and liquids; assisting in feeding those in need of help; taking vital signs and reporting abnormal findings; and participating actively in all routine hygiene procedures related to resident care.

PHYSICIAN ASSISTANTS   The physician assistant (PA), under the supervision of a physician, performs diagnostic, therapeutic, preventive, and health maintenance services. Working as members of the healthcare team, PAs take medical histories, examine patients, order and interpret laboratory reports and x-rays, and make diagnoses. They also treat minor injuries by suturing, splinting, and casting. PAs record progress notes, instruct and counsel patients, and order or carry out therapy. In almost every state, PAs may prescribe medications.

PHARMACISTS   Hospital pharmacists monitor a patient's drug therapy, prepare intravenous medications and feedings, oversee drug administration, and make purchasing decisions. Pharmacists are important members of many healthcare teams.

SOCIAL WORKERS   The field of social work is incredibly broad. A bachelor of arts in social work is always required; a master's degree in social work (MSW) is increasingly required. The undergraduate degree is broad-based, with elective courses in substance abuse, grief, and race and gender issues. Graduate programs explore human behavior, mental disorders, and methods of intervention and psychotherapy in greater depth.

CHIROPRACTORS   A doctor of chiropractic (DC) has completed a minimum of 2 years of college credit toward a baccalaureate degree and 3 to 4 years at a chiropractic college. Chiropractic emphasizes a holistic approach to health and is based on the premise that the relationship between structure and function in the human body (particularly of the spinal column and nervous system) is a significant health factor. Chiropractors believe that when the spinal column is out of alignment the body's natural defenses against disease and illness are lowered. Chiropractors realign the spinal column so that the body stays in a state of homeostasis, or balance.

PHYSICAL THERAPISTS   Physical therapists design and administer rehabilitative exercise programs for people with injuries or disabilities that affect their daily functioning.

ATHLETIC TRAINERS   Athletic trainers provide services such as injury prevention, recognition, immediate care, treatment, and rehabilitation of athletic trauma.

OCCUPATIONAL THERAPISTS   Occupational therapists and their assistants provide service to individuals whose abilities to cope with the tasks of living are threatened or impaired by developmental deficits, the aging process, poverty and cultural differences, physical injury or illness, or psychological and social disability. The therapy is directed toward teaching adaptive skills and enhancing performance capacity to achieve optimal function, prevent disability, or maintain health. The goal is the highest possible functional independence for self-care, work, and leisure.

SPEECH-LANGUAGE PATHOLOGISTS   Speech-language pathologists assess, diagnose, treat, and help prevent speech, language, cognitive, communication, voice, swallowing, and fluency problems. Specifically related to dietetics, speech-language pathologists work with people who have oral motor problems that cause eating and swallowing difficulties.

MEDICAL LABORATORY TECHNICIANS/TECHNOLOGISTS   Under the supervision of a pathologist, a "lab tech" performs lab tests, using precision instruments on blood, tissues, and body fluids to detect, diagnose, and treat diseases. Medical lab technologists are able to perform the same duties as a technician and can also perform more complex analyses, discrimination, and detection of errors. Histologic technicians/technologists specialize in the preparation of body tissues for laboratory analysis.

RADIOLOGIC TECHNOLOGISTS   Under the supervision of radiation oncologists, "rad techs" administer radiation therapy to patients. Radiographers, also under the supervision of qualified physicians, provide patient service using imaging modalities.

NUCLEAR MEDICINE TECHNOLOGISTS   A nuclear medicine technologist assists a nuclear medicine physician. These physicians use the nuclear properties of radioactive and stable nuclides to make diagnostic evaluations of the anatomic or physiologic conditions of the body.

RESPIRATORY THERAPISTS   The respiratory therapist and respiratory therapy technician evaluate all data to determine the appropriate respiratory care for a patient and conduct the therapeutic procedures to carry out this plan.

Medical Assistants

Medical assistants assist physicians in their offices or other medical settings by performing a variety of administrative and clinical duties.

MEDICAL RECORDS ADMINISTRATORS   A medical record comprises the complete and permanent documents maintained for every person treated in a medical facility. Medical records administrators manage the medical record in compliance with medical, administrative, ethical, and legal requirements. The medical records technician (MRT) is responsible for maintaining the medical records.

Summary

Management guru Ken Blanchard wisely observed, "None of us is as smart as all of us." Teamwork is important in the healthcare professions today, partly because of the enormous number of people employed in these careers. The team approach is an effective way of dealing with the fragmentation of care that may occur because of specialization.

Teamwork may be problematic if roles are not clearly defined, communication is not adequate and open, members fail to be good team players, and team goals are not clearly defined. Accurate and timely sharing of data is a key element in the effectiveness of the team effort. Team conferences, in which all team members share information and participate in decision making, are the preferred approach.

Dietitians, dietetic technicians, and dietary managers are the members of the dietetic team. They have all received formal training in foods and nutrition, and, as a team, they work in a wide variety of settings. Dietitians, who are recognized experts in food and nutrition, are found working in the business, clinical, community, consulting, education, management, and research arenas. Dietetic technicians must complete a 2-year associate degree in an Academy of Nutrition and Dietetics–approved dietetic technician program and then pass the registration examination for dietetic technicians. Dietary managers complete a 1-year college course.

Effective teamwork requires shared goals, clearly defined roles, and a plan for coordinating efforts. Whenever possible, the patient should be part of the team. Any health professional can testify to the importance of patient cooperation in the diagnostic, therapeutic, and rehabilitative processes.

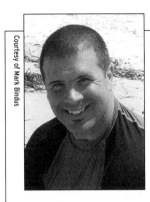

Profile of a Professional

Mark Bindus, RD, LD

Director of Food Services and Wellness
Twinsburg City Schools
Twinsburg, Ohio

Education:
BS in Nutrition and Dietetics, University of Akron, Akron, Ohio
Coordinated Program in Dietetics

How did you first hear about dietetics and decide to become a Registered Dietitian?

I started out in college as a communications major. After 1½ years, I decided that because of my interest in sports and bodybuilding, I would enjoy working in sports nutrition, and thus I headed toward dietetics.

Where did you do your supervised practice experience in your Coordinated Program?

During the last 2 years of the CP program, I interned at Akron General Medical Center, Akron City Hospital, Mercy Medical Center, and North Royalton City Schools.

Are you involved in professional organizations?

I am a member of the Academy of Nutrition and Dietetics, the Ohio Dietetic Association, the School Nutrition Association, and Building Healthy Kids at Akron Children's Hospital, as well as being Wellness Coordinator for Twinsburg City Schools. I'm really proud that our schools were recognized with a Gold Medal in the Buckeye Best Healthy Schools competition, a program designed to recognize those schools whose policies and practices reflect a high priority on healthy outcomes for children.

Briefly describe your career path in dietetics. What are you doing now?

When I first began the Coordinated Program in dietetics, my plan was to finish the program, get my registration, and then go back to school to get my masters in exercise physiology so that I could pursue a job working with professional athletes. This path led me to take a supervised practice placement at North Royalton City Schools, where I had several opportunities to teach student athletes about proper sports nutrition. Although I did enjoy that opportunity, what I discovered was that I really enjoyed the management end of dietetics and the creative part of recipe development and menu planning.

Seventeen years later, I still enjoy what I do. As District Dietitian of Twinsburg City Schools, I am also the Wellness Coordinator, creating and maintaining my own web page, hiring, managing, and evaluating employees, and projecting and controlling the budget, as well as occasionally getting into the classrooms to teach nutrition. As I tell dietetic students, working in school foodservice provides me the opportunity to actually impact students' health by pushing them to try new, healthful foods. Over the last number of years, our foodservice has changed over to whole-grain breads and pizza crusts, whole-wheat pastas, brown rice, dark green salads (romaine and spinach), and an assortment of fresh fruits and vegetables that are all offered on a daily basis. We eliminated pop, Gatorade, and juice drinks and got rid of all the high-fat, high-sugar vending items over 6 years ago, and we are always making changes to improve our offerings nutritionally.

What excites you about dietetics and the future of our profession?

I believe that as a country we are finally getting to the place where everyone wants to know a little more about how they can improve their health by what they eat. This really gives us the opportunity to step forward and show that we are the experts.

Why/how is teamwork important to you in your position? How have you been involved in team projects?

As the District Dietitian for Twinsburg City Schools, every new thing that we implement is done using a team approach. My employees are the most essential part of the process, and their input is invaluable, because they will be the ones to actually "do" whatever is needed to make a change work.

What words of wisdom do you have for future dietetics professionals?
Never rule out working in any particular area in dietetics. All through college I always said that I would never work in foodservice, and here I am today, 17 years later—all in school foodservice, and I wouldn't change a thing. Not only do I love the work that I do, but I also enjoy the perks that go with working for schools: no weekends, getting spring and winter breaks, a month off in the summer, and great benefits!

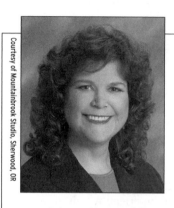

Courtesy of Mountainbrook Studio, Sherwood, OR

Profile of a Professional

Gretchen Vannice, MS, RD

Managing Director
Omega-3 RD Nutrition Consulting
Portland, Oregon

Education:
BS in Nutrition, Oregon State University, Corvallis, Oregon
MS in Nutritional Science, San Jose State University,
  San Jose, California
Dietetic Internship, San Jose State University, San Jose,
  California

How did you first hear about dietetics and decide to become a Registered Dietitian?
I became keenly interested in nutrition after taking a class my second year in college. I became a Registered Dietitian after graduate school because I saw the value in completing the dietetic internship and I wanted to work in health care.

What are some examples of your professional involvement?
In undergraduate and graduate school, I was involved in the local dietetics organizations. In graduate school, I represented the state dietetics group in legislative events and co-coordinated the annual continuing education conference. It was an awesome experience and still on my résumé today. I've been a member of the American Dietetic Association, now known as the Academy of Nutrition and Dietetics, since graduate school. After I became registered, I joined the Dietitians in Integrative Medicine Dietetics Practice Group (DPG). I volunteered to coordinate the continuing education program for the nationwide group for 3 years, and then served on the Executive Board for 2 years. I've remained a member and continue to support the group. The greatest benefit has been being in touch with colleagues who share similar interests.

Have you received honors or awards?
In 2007, I received the Excellence in Practice Award from the Dietitians in Integrative Medicine DPG for dedication and contribution to dietetics professionals. In 2009, I presented the First Annual William E. Connor, MD Memorial Lecture at Oregon State Health Sciences University.

Briefly describe your career path in dietetics. What are you doing now?
I worked as a health educator at Kaiser Permanente Medical Center, managing the Weight Management and Tobacco Cessation programs. Because I was the only RD in the department, I was the nutrition resource for the Diabetes, Women's Health, and HIV/AIDs programs as well. I have always had an interest in evidence-based natural products and integrative medicine, so I left Kaiser when I was offered a position in research and development for a dietary supplement company. I have worked in management with research, education, and training for dietary supplements. When the last company I worked for was sold, I started a consulting business.

What excites you about dietetics and the future of our profession?
As a nation, we are beginning to wake up to the power and importance of nutrition and preventive health. Waiting until people get sick before intervening never made

sense to me. Whether it is food, fish oil, or ginger root, some natural products have health benefits, and some do not; research will show the way. This is an area for dietitians to be keenly aware of the science and stay close to the evidence.

Why/how is teamwork important to you in your position? How have you been involved in team projects?
I would not have employment today without teamwork. As a consultant, my work comes through relationships I have built during my career. In addition, I am chair of the International Science Committee for the Global Organization for Omega-3 EPA and DHA and sit on the executive board of the International Omega-3 Consortium for Health and Medicine. The camaraderie I've developed, the excitement in sharing science, and the professional exposure from both of these volunteer positions is remarkable, and just fun.

What words of wisdom do you have for future dietetics professionals?
People will take you and our profession as seriously as you take yourself. Don't sell yourself short. Know your worth. Other healthcare professionals do not have your depth of knowledge in food or applied nutrition science. There are a myriad of people calling themselves nutrition professionals with little to no training, and/or no valid credentials. RDs are exceptionally well trained, well skilled, and better prepared; remember that. And volunteering has been invaluable. Your career is what you make it. Everyone likes food. Enjoy the path.

Suggested Activities

1. Find out what's new with teams and teamwork. Teams are becoming an increasingly more important part of organizational life, and, as a result, much is changing in this area. Go to the *Fast Company* website at www .fastcompany.com. Click the "Magazine" main menu tab on the homepage. On the Magazine page, type "teamwork" into the Search box. Select and read at least two of the full-text articles and find at least three good ideas for successful teamwork. Share these with your classmates.

2. How good a team player are you? Could you become a better team player? Which of your teamwork skills need improvement? Think of a team you are currently on or a team you may have been on in the past and take the quiz at www.mindtools.com. Were you surprised by the results? How will this self-knowledge be of help to you in forming or working on a team?

3. Want to improve your teamwork or communication skills? Go to www.gamesforgroups.com, under the Therapeutic Games tab, click the "Teamwork Games" or the "Communication Games" links. Gather the materials needed. With a group of classmates, try some of the teamwork and communication exercises.

4. Contact a large medical center or hospital in your area to see whether it has a dietetic team. Talk to the members of the team to determine their roles and responsibilities in delivering nutritional care to clients.

5. With a team of fellow students, write a paper on the principles of teamwork. In doing the research and writing the paper, apply the principles that have been found to be effective. Evaluate your success as a team. What worked well and why? What didn't work and why?

6. Choose any of the allied health professions. Do an in-depth study of its educational requirements, job responsibilities, areas of specialization, and so on.

7. Visit a local hospital cafeteria, and talk to as many of its employees as you can. Try to determine if, how, and to what extent they work with members of the dietetic team.

8. Volunteer to work in a hospital or other healthcare facility. This is an excellent way to learn about various healthcare professions and to help those who need it at the same time.

9. Are you interested in the salaries offered for the different allied health professions? The Bureau of Labor Statistics gathers employment and wage data periodically and reports it on its website. Go to www.bls.gov and compare the wage estimates shown. Which states and metropolitan areas offer the highest salaries?

10. Are you a good communicator? Communication is such an everyday activity that it is seldom given much thought. This activity is an opportunity to assess your communication style and skills to see how you might become a more effective communicator. Visit the website www.queendom.com. Click the main menu category "Tests." Under "Relationship Tests," click "Interpersonal Communication Skills Test." Were you surprised by the results? What are your strengths and limitations, and what do you need to do to improve?

Selected Websites

- www.aapa.org—American Academy of Physician Assistants
- www.ama-assn.org—American Medical Association
- www.bls.gov—U.S. Bureau of Labor Statistics
- www.fastcompany.com—Site features full-text magazine articles on teamwork and team building
- www.gamesforgroups.com—Site features therapeutic and team-building games
- www.mindtools.com—Site features a quiz to assess team effectiveness
- www.osteopathic.org—American Osteopathic Association
- www.queendom.com—Site offers a variety of online tests
- www.teambuildersplus.com—Team Builders Plus helps individuals develop the skills to create a team environment

Suggested Readings

Damp DV. *Health Care Job Explosion! High Growth Health Care Careers and Job Locator.* 3rd ed. Moon Township, PA: Bookhaven Press LLC; 2001.

Fazio Maruca R. What makes teams work. *Fast Company.* October 31, 2000. http://www.fastcompany.com/41112/what-makes-teams-work. Accessed February 18, 2013.

Fishman C. The Whole Foods recipe for teamwork. *Fast Company.* April 31, 1996. Available at: http://www.fastcompany.com/26641/whole-foods-recipe-teamwork. Accessed February 18, 2013.

Kouzes JM, Posner BZ. *The Leadership Challenge*, 4th ed. San Francisco: Jossey-Bass; 2007.

Levi D. *Group Dynamics for Teams*. Thousand Oaks, CA: Sage; 2001.

Moores S. Six heads are better than one. *ADA Times* 2003;1(1):1–3.

Roberts P. The agenda—total teamwork. *Fast Company*. March 31, 1999. http://www.fastcompany.com/36969/agenda-total-teamwork. Accessed February 18, 2013.

Stanfield P, Hui YH. *Introduction to the Health Professions*. Sudbury, MA. Jones and Bartlett Publishers; 1998.

References

1. Reprinted from Journal of the American Dietetic Association, 96, Number 12 (December 1996), George I. Balch, "Employers' Perceptions of the Roles of Dietetics Practitioners: Challenges to Survive and Opportunities to Thrive," pp. 1301–1305, Copyright 1996, with permission from Elsevier.

2. The Association of Schools of Allied Health Professions. Available at: http://www.asahp.org. Accessed January 28, 2004.

3. Lumsden G, Lumsden D. *Communicating in Groups and Teams: Sharing Leadership*. Belmont, CA: Wadsworth; 2000.

4. Spear BA, Sturdevant M, Boutelle K. The Team Approach to Treatment of Adolescents with Eating Disorders. Presentation at Food & Nutrition Conference & Expo, American Dietetic Association. October 2003.

5. Katzenbach J, Smith D. *The Wisdom of Teams*. Boston: Harvard Business School Press; 1993:45.

6. Healthy Iowans 2010 Planning Process—Roles for Key Actors. Available at: http://www.phf.org/Hptools/state/keyactors.pdf. Accessed January 28, 2004.

7. Kreitner R. *Management*, 9th ed. Boston: Houghton Mifflin; 2004.

8. Cartwright D, Zander A. *Group Dynamics: Research and Theory*, 3rd ed. New York: HarperCollins; 1968.

9. Ashforth B, Kreiner GE, Fugate M. All in a day's work: boundaries and micro role transitions. *Acad Manage Rev.* 2000;25:472–491.

10. Chatman JA, Flynn FJ. The influence of demographic heterogeneity on the emergence and consequences of cooperative norms in work teams. *Acad Manage J.* 2001;44:956–974.

11. Feldman DC. The development and enforcement of group norms. *Acad Manage Rev.* 1984;9:47–53.

12. Jewell LN, Reitz HJ. *Group Effectiveness in Organizations*. Glenview, IL: Scott, Foresman and Company; 1983:15–20.

13. Payne-Palacio J, Theis M. *Introduction to Foodservice*, 11th ed. Upper Saddle River, NJ: Prentice Hall; 2010.

14. House A, Dallinger JM, Kilgallen D. Androgyny and rhetorical sensitivity: the connection of gender and communicator style. *Commun Rep.* 1998:11;12–19.

15. Satir V. Making contact. In: Stewart J, ed. *Bridges Not Walls*, 5th ed. New York: McGraw-Hill; 1990.

16. Waldron VR, Applegate JL. Person-centered tactics during verbal disagreements: effects on student perceptions of persuasiveness and social attraction. *Commun Ed.* 1998;47:53–66.

17. Watzlawick P, Beavin JH, Jackson DD. *Pragmatics of Human Communication*. New York: Norton; 1967.

18. Thamhain HJ. Managing technologically innovative team efforts toward new product success. *J Prod Innovation Manage.* 1990;7:5–18.

19. U.S. Department of Labor. Bureau of Labor Statistics. *Occupational Outlook Handbook*. Available at: http://www.bls.gov. Accessed January 28, 2004.

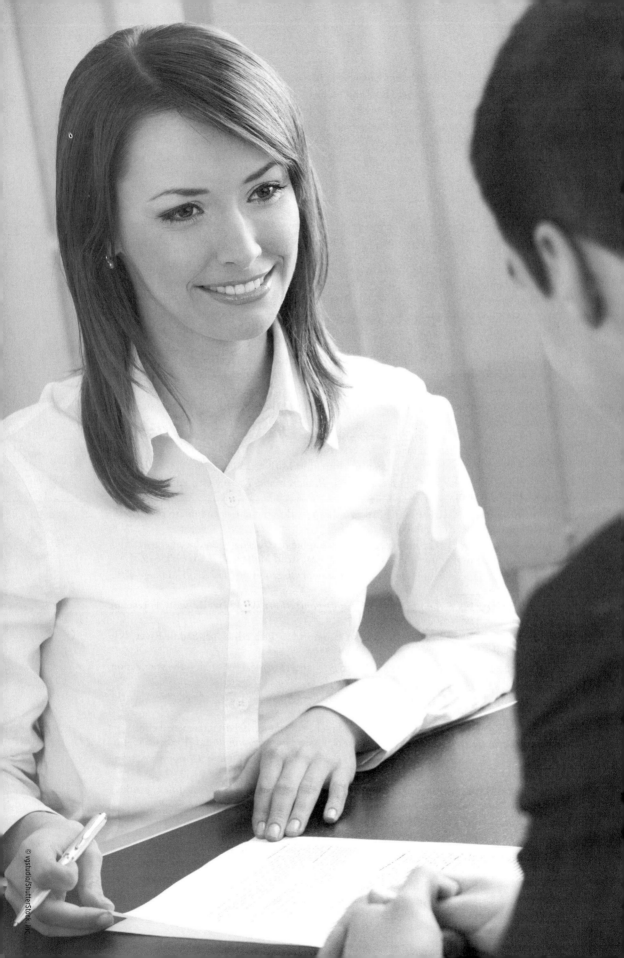

Beginning Your Path to Success in Dietetics

Who Are You?

Your path to success in any chosen profession begins with a bit of self-knowledge. What are your interests, strengths, and weaknesses? What are your short- and long-term goals? Where do you want to go, and how do you expect to get there? Some students are fortunate enough to have decided on their career goals by the time they begin college, but many others remain undecided.

This chapter focuses on some professional tools that will help you to answer some of the questions posed above. SWOT analysis and portfolios are useful self-assessment tools for determining your strengths, weaknesses, areas of interest, and goals. Then, a good résumé and strong interview skills will help you get where you want to go.

The Portfolio

Once only carried by artists, models, and photographers, the portfolio has now become almost the norm for professionals in today's competitive job market. In fact, the dietetic profession's accreditation committee now requires a professional development portfolio as a part of the continuing education program for registered dietitians. This portfolio is discussed in greater detail in Chapter 7. The portfolios discussed in this chapter—the student portfolio and the career portfolio—are of a more personal nature and will be useful to you before you reach the registration requirement stage. In fact, these portfolios are important tools for life. Always a work in progress, your portfolios should change and grow with you. New skills will be refined and demonstrated, new work experiences will be added, the number of work samples will grow and expand, and your goals and philosophy may shift and evolve to higher levels.

What is a portfolio? A *portfolio* may be defined as a coherent (not exhaustive) set of materials, including work samples and reflective statements on these samples, compiled by a person to represent his or her practice as related to desired outcomes. Some think of it as a much-expanded form of a résumé. More practically speaking, a portfolio is a collection of items organized in a notebook. Collecting these items throughout your college career helps you to recognize skills and abilities you possess in relation to your goals. Later, the portfolio can be used to market your qualifications for an internship or to an employer after graduation.

A portfolio is a powerful tool, not so much because of the product, but because of the process required to create it. The process takes time and thought. It is a complex, thought-provoking exercise in self-evaluation—reflection, decision making, and goal setting—that takes place over time. The product is important, too. The portfolio is a unique and valuable means of communication between you and others. Potential employers, internship directors, teachers, and career counselors all may benefit from reading your portfolio. A sense of accomplishment, self-satisfaction, and pride is possible because your portfolio is a display of your individual goals, growth, and achievement, as well as a testimony to acquired knowledge and professional and personal attributes.

What Are the Purposes of a Portfolio?

Portfolios serve many purposes. The focus in this chapter is on portfolios that will initially be used for self-assessment and evaluation, to record and display professional goals, growth, and achievement. Later in your career, the professional development portfolio for maintaining registration will serve as a foundation for career-long, self-directed professional development.

Developing a portfolio in college will help you to evaluate yourself and your career decisions. Interests that are documented in your portfolio can be matched to possible careers. You can also compare the skill level displayed in your portfolio to the level needed in your chosen career. A student portfolio allows you to:

- Think about and plan your future
- Evaluate your progress
- Identify learning experiences that will help you reach your goals
- Demonstrate what you know and can do
- Learn to use a progressive tool that will be carried forward from year to year to recognize vital pieces of your personal, academic, and career development process
- Record ongoing work and accomplishments

After college graduation, your portfolio may be used to obtain an internship or job or it may follow you to graduate school. The portfolio allows you to demonstrate examples of work you have done and your accomplishments. Keep in mind that the portfolio should be used judiciously to support points you make verbally in an interview regarding your experience, skills, or accomplishments. Portfolios are not yet mandatory in employment interviews, but they are increasingly welcomed, and there is reason to believe that in the future they will be requested.

A portfolio also allows you to:

- Have an edge in the promotion process
- Shine in a performance review
- Distinguish yourself from the competition
- Turn a job interview into an offer
- Find the right position for you
- Create the opportunity to stand out
- Be professionally empowered
- Possess better, more authentic, more robust evidence of good practice—for reflection, discussion, and/or evaluation
- Leave a legacy to new members of the profession

Where Do I Start?

Your portfolio is all about making plans. The portfolio-creation process includes five steps: reflection, assessment, planning, implementation, and evaluation.

Step 1: Reflection. This first step is the most important and possibly the most difficult. The more thought you put into this step, the more rewarding your portfolio will be. The questions to ask and answer are:

- What are my strengths, weaknesses, and interests?
- What do I enjoy most in my coursework, work experiences, etc.?
- What are my short- and long-term professional and personal goals?

Answers to these questions should be written out and included in the portfolio. You may want to write a personal statement or reflective autobiography, a story of your intellectual, emotional, and spiritual growth told by the person who knows it best—you. It requires some very deep reflective thought and should work to reveal to you some new insights into who, why, where, and what you are at the present time.

Step 2: Assessment. Based on your short- and long-term goals and perceived weaknesses, what are your learning needs? Prioritize these needs based on their level of importance in reaching your goals. This step may help you to determine which classes would make good electives and what work experience would help to get you accepted to the internship of your choice.

Step 3: Planning. What is needed to accomplish your learning needs? Each learning need should relate to at least one goal, and that learning need should be accomplished with a proposed plan.

Step 4: Implementation. Put the plan into motion. Document what you are doing or have done to accomplish your plans. A very valuable addition to a portfolio is "work in progress."

Step 5: Evaluation. Review your progress over the past few years. Evaluate what you have learned and how you have applied the new knowledge. Revise your goals as they are accomplished, writing new goals as some are achieved.

What Should I Include in My Student Portfolio?

The answer to this question is not easy. One answer is "it depends on the purpose and the audience." Still, there are some general guidelines and suggestions for what to include. First, keep in mind that a portfolio is representative, not comprehensive. Everything chosen should represent a significant aspect of you and/or your work. Second, because the primary purpose of the student and career portfolios is self-assessment, a reflective statement should accompany each item that is included in them. The final point to keep in mind is that a portfolio is a work in progress and that anything included may be later deleted or added as is fitting to your professional development. Possible items to include are:

Community/Club Activities
- Certificate of participation in a program
- Evaluation written by a supervisor or other person with whom you have worked or studied
- Outline of a plan you designed to lead a program or presentation
- Pictures of members participating in an event you helped to plan
- Special notes or feedback for your help with a project
- Invitations/program/poster designed for a special event
- Records (nonconfidential) you maintained for accuracy
- Agenda describing items discussed in a committee in which you were involved
- Sketch of a layout used to determine setup of equipment and facilities for an event
- Record of the sales you achieved for fund-raising

Classroom/School Experiences
- Examples of assignments with special comments from the faculty member
- Examples of works in progress or various stages of a project
- Actual item or picture of the item created through a class project
- Report on a topic of special interest
- Outline of a memorable presentation to a class
- Transcripts of grades highlighting the classes you most enjoyed
- Certificate of completion of class or assignment
- Copy of a letter written to a person you were required to contact for a class assignment
- Pictures or souvenirs from a place to which you traveled for a field trip (**Figure 4–1**) or for study abroad
- Positive evaluation received from a faculty member or supervisor
- Summary of a research project you designed

Academic Recognition
- Letter or certificate that recognizes you as a scholarship recipient
- Letter or certificate that designates you as achieving the Dean's List
- Graduation program highlighting designation as valedictorian, salutatorian, or special honoree
- Summary of scholarly research project and/or results
- Newspaper article noting recognition of special honors

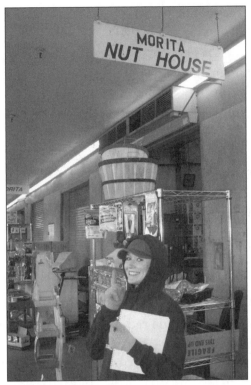

FIGURE 4–1 A dietetic student has fun on an early morning field trip to the Los Angeles Wholesale Produce Market.
Courtesy of Lari Bright

- Extracurricular activities
- Special awards for participation in an event
- Trophies/ribbons for winning or placing in a competition
- Newspaper clippings of individual or team accomplishments
- Pictures of team or individual participation in an event
- Letters or commendation from a coach, advisor, or other individuals associated with athletic achievement

Special Skills
- Examples of handouts, letters, memos, reports, charts, graphs, brochures, and so on using computer software or program languages
- Correspondence written in a foreign language or documentation of a study abroad or foreign exchange program
- Evidence of a hobby, craft, or topic of special interest, or certification of skill level such as Water Safety instructor, First Aid, or CPR
- Skill sets (groups of skills in a particular area, such as expertise with various software programs)

Work Related
- Letters of recommendation from present or former employers
- Performance evaluations
- Special recognitions from supervisor or customer for work performed

- Employee-of-the-month award
- Clippings from employee newsletter relating to you

Other

- Statement of originality and confidentiality (a brief statement indicating that the portfolio is your work and should not be copied without permission)
- Philosophy statement (a brief description of your beliefs about yourself and the profession)
- Academic plan of study (your plan of study that lists courses you have taken to fulfill your degree)
- Your résumé and cover letter
- Personal statement/reflective autobiography
- Career summary and goals
- List of awards and honors
- List of conferences and workshops in which you have participated
- Academic transcripts, degrees, and qualifications
- References and contact details of references

The choice of what to include requires careful decision making. Asking the following questions may help:

1. What do I want my portfolio to show about me? What are my attributes?
2. What do I want my portfolio to demonstrate about me as a learner? How and what have I learned?
3. What directions for my future growth and development does my self-evaluation suggest? How can I show these in my portfolio?
4. What points have others made about me as a student? How can I show them in my portfolio?
5. What effect does my work experience have on me? How can I show this in my portfolio?
6. What overall impression do I want my portfolio to give a reader about me as a learner?

Turn Your Student Portfolio into a Career Portfolio

Toward the end of your college career, it is time to make some slight adjustments in the contents of your student portfolio. A SWOT analysis should be included. SWOT stands for strengths, weaknesses, opportunities, and threats (**Figure 4–2**). You can use a SWOT analysis to focus your self-assessment in order to make better decisions about your future. Understanding your strengths and weaknesses and the opportunities available to you and the threats you might face will enable you to utilize your talents, manage your weaknesses, uncover and take advantage of opportunities, and eliminate threats.

Using the worksheet, begin by writing down your strengths and weaknesses. Ask others for their opinions; be honest, objective, and realistic. Consider skills related to your career goals, teamwork, communication,

SWOT Analysis Worksheet

Internal Factors

Your Strengths What do you do well? What do others see as your strengths? Where do you excel when compared to others?	**Your Weaknesses** What could you improve? What do others see as your weaknesses? What would make you a better practioner?
Opportunities What good opportunities are available to you? What trends could you take advantage of? Which of your strengths could you turn into opportunities?	**Threats** What trends could you harm you? What competition do you face? Which of your weaknesses expose you to potential threats?

POSITIVES (left side) — **NEGATIVES** (right side)

External Factors

FIGURE 4–2 A SWOT analysis worksheet.

and technology. Also consider your personal and social skills. For your strengths, consider the questions posed on the form. Also think about which of your achievements make you most proud. In addition to the questions on the form relating to weaknesses, what tasks do you tend to avoid because of a lack of confidence in doing them? What are your negative work habits and personality traits? Strengths and weaknesses are internal factors because they are under your control.

Opportunities and threats are external factors because you do not control them. However, you can use your strengths to take advantage of opportunities. Is there a need in the field that no one is filling? Would eliminating any of your weaknesses open up new opportunities for you? In terms of threats, what obstacles do you face in reaching your goals? How can these threats be managed or eliminated?

In addition to the SWOT analysis, the student portfolio needs to be updated and contents selected for the change in purpose and audience. As shown in **Figure 4–3**, the career portfolio is used for self-assessment as well as for obtaining a position, an internship, admission to graduate school, or a promotion. The contents of the career portfolio are a good starting point for the professional development portfolio that will be required to maintain registered status.

The Matter of Style

Presentation and organization are important aspects of your portfolio. Three-ring binders, artists' portfolio cases, and zippered leather cases are good options to hold portfolio contents. Clear plastic, three-hole-punched pockets hold documents and work samples, protect the materials, and give the portfolio a professional look. A table of contents and tabs improve readability. Extra-wide three-ring tabs with labels are necessary for the tabs to show when using sheet protectors. Photo sheet holders are available to hold pictures and provide spaces for typed captions. Zippered pouches and CD and diskette holders should be used if videos, CDs, or diskettes are included. Every document should have a caption that leads the reader to the importance of the piece and a reflective statement. A reflective statement is simply your thoughts about the work (**Figure 4–4**).

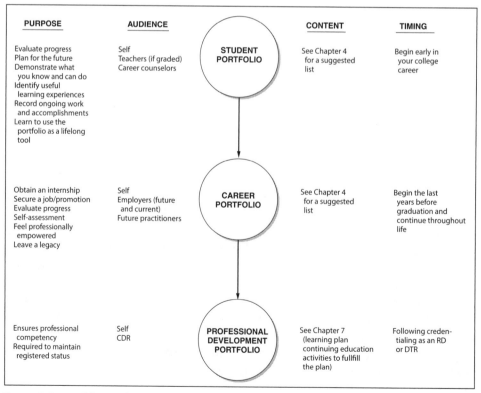

PURPOSE	AUDIENCE		CONTENT	TIMING

Evaluate progress
Plan for the future
Demonstrate what
  you know and can do
Identify useful
  learning experiences
Record ongoing work
  and accomplishments
Learn to use the
  portfolio as a lifelong
  tool
	Self
	Teachers (if graded)
	Career counselors
		STUDENT
		PORTFOLIO
			See Chapter 4
			for a suggested
			list
				Begin early in
				  your college
				  career

Obtain an internship
Secure a job/promotion
Evaluate progress
Self-assessment
Feel professionally
  empowered
Leave a legacy
	Self
	Employers (future
	  and current)
	Future practitioners
		CAREER
		PORTFOLIO
			See Chapter 4
			for a suggested
			list
				Begin the last
				  years before
				  graduation and
				  continue throughout
				  life

Ensures professional
  competency
Required to maintain
  registered status
	Self
	CDR
		PROFESSIONAL
		DEVELOPMENT
		PORTFOLIO
			See Chapter 7
			(learning plan
			continuing education
			activities to fullfill
			the plan)
				Following creden-
				  tialing as an RD
				  or DTR

Figure 4–3 A portfolio timeline.

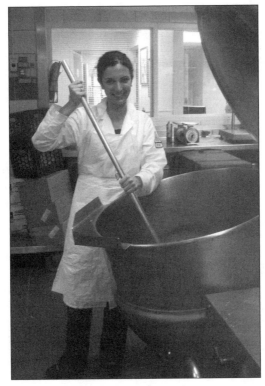

FIGURE 4–4 A dietetic intern gets hands-on experience in quantity food production.
Courtesy of Michele Coelho, RD

These thoughts might include the answers to such questions as "What did I learn from doing it?" "How would I do it differently the next time?" and "Why did I receive the grade I did?"

Avoid using anything handwritten (with the exception of an instructor's handwritten comments on an assignment or notes from others), paper clips, staples, or tape. These detract from the professional look. Proofread everything carefully, and be consistent in margins, tabs, and font style. Allow for some white space on each page and use bullet points for added emphasis, conciseness, and readability.

Once you have gathered your materials, sorting, choosing, and organizing come next. Sort your materials into small clusters, such as class projects, writing samples, team efforts, projects demonstrating organization and professionalism, and so on. Choose from the small clusters based on which items show the most skills and competencies, which are most interesting to you, which demonstrate your best work, and which relate most to your goals. Organize the chosen samples into a logical sequence. One possible order might be:

- Table of Contents
- Statement of originality and confidentiality
- Personal philosophy statement and goals
- Résumé
- Work samples and skill sets

- List of works in progress
- Certificates, diplomas, and degrees
- Samples of community service
- Professional memberships and samples of service
- Academic plan of study
- Faculty and employer biographies
- List of references

What About an Electronic Portfolio?

Electronic portfolios are typically designed as web pages that are posted to an Internet location or burned onto a CD. They may be used as a supplement to the hard-copy version or stand alone. An electronic portfolio can be an extraordinarily powerful tool, but it must have a professional appearance and be easy to navigate. The visual impact can be quite striking. It is possible to use photos, sound, animation, and even streaming video. Having an electronic portfolio demonstrates to others that you are technically savvy, current, and contemporary. It gives interviewers an opportunity to get further information about you either before or after the interview.

The Résumé

A résumé is simply a marketing tool that outlines your skills and experiences so that someone can see at a glance how you might fit in a position. This decision is often made in less than 30 seconds. So your résumé needs to be succinct, organized, and clearly focused on the particular purpose for which it is being used. To provide more information to the interviewer, the statement "Portfolio Available on Request" may be included at the bottom of your résumé.

Your résumé is also an example of your writing, communication, and organizational skills. The content, format, and style of your résumé and the accompanying cover letter are all very important details, and each is covered in the following sections.

Content

Content should **focus on relevant accomplishments and skills, not job duties and responsibilities**. A way to ensure this focus is to use project–action–results (PAR) statements when describing your school and work experiences. For example:

Project—Conducted research project on sanitation of university foodservice cutting boards.

Action—Designed and conducted the experiment.

Result—Determined best method for sanitation of cutting boards; reported results to the foodservice contractor, who implemented the method.

Where possible, quantify your experiences to convey the size or scale of projects, budgets, and/or results to make a stronger impression. Numbers, percentages, and dollars stand out in the body of a résumé. For example, rather than "Served as president of the Student Nutrition and Dietetics Association," say "Presided over 50-member Student Nutrition and Dietetics Association that resulted in five projects and nine activities (50% increase over last year)."

Include only relevant information by choosing, prioritizing, and tailoring headings and experience to the position for which you are applying. For example:

Objective—Dietetic Internship

Diet Office Experience (not Work Experience) (**Figure 4–5**)

To add life to your résumé, use bulleted sentences that begin with action words like *prepared, presented, developed*, and *monitored*. A formula for building a résumé entry is:

Action Verb(s) + Object/Person + to/for whom OR

of/on/from/in what OR

by/through/with what

For example:

Organized group activities in a nursing home

Answered questions on diet at campus health fair

For each job listing, ask yourself "Of which accomplishment in this position am I most proud?"

List your strengths first, where they will be most likely to be read. Rather than going into depth in any one area, use your résumé to highlight your breadth of knowledge. The interview and portfolio can then provide more detail. At all times, be honest about your skills and work experiences.

Do not include any data related to salary expectations, religious or political affiliations, geographical restrictions, age, or relationship status. Include GPA only if it is 3.0 or above.

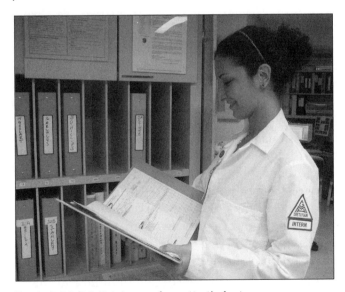

FIGURE 4–5 A dietetic intern reads a patient's chart.
Courtesy of Michele Coelho, RD

Content headings might include any and all of the following:

- Personal Contact Information: name, address, phone, email, website
- Objective/Summary of Qualifications
- Education and Training
- Relevant Courses/Projects
- Scholarships/Awards
- Work Experience
- Relevant Skills Section
- Accomplishments/Professional Achievements
- Relevant Presentations/Publications
- Professional Affiliations
- Activities/Interests

Some experts suggest that an initial impression can be made with a résumé that begins with a profile rather than the standard objective statement. A well-written profile provides a summary of your skills and identifies your unique qualities and strengths. To write a profile, consider these questions:

Who am I?

What do I like to do?

What are my skills and abilities?

What type of work have I done in the past?

What type of work would I like to do in the future?

An example of a profile statement would be "A hard-working, energetic dietetic student who will graduate from a rigorous nutritional science program this year; experienced in hospital dietetics, undergraduate research, and working on team projects; a self-starter with a unique flair for multitasking, planning and organizing assignments, and working with people."

Format

There are basically three formats to choose from: reverse chronological, functional, and combination.

The reverse chronological résumé. This format is the most commonly used, most widely accepted, most familiar to employers, and easiest to read. Work experiences are listed in chronological order starting with the most recent and working back through the years. The reverse chronological format is particularly effective when:

- You have professional experience in the field of interest
- You have held impressive job titles and/or have worked for highly regarded employers within your targeted field
- You have progressed into positions in the field with more responsibility
- You have changed jobs and fields of work frequently
- You want to change your field of work to something different from your past work experience
- You want to highlight your skills

The functional résumé. This format became popular in the 1970s and 1980s and is viewed skeptically by some employers. It places emphasis on your qualifications without focus on specific dates. The functional résumé summarizes your professional functions or experiences and avoids or minimizes your employment history. For example, this format would include headings such as "teaching skills," "management skills," and "patient relations skills." Each skill area is then illustrated by listing experiences that demonstrate that skill. This format is particularly effective when:

- You are a recent graduate without a lot of professional experience in the field, but you have relevant coursework and training
- You want to emphasize skills you possess that have not been used in recent work experiences
- You are changing careers (because the format outlines transferable work skills)
- You are a returning employee after an absence from the workforce or you are an older worker (because dates are minimized)

It is particularly *ineffective* when:

- You do not have a lot of time to create your résumé (it is more difficult to write)
- You want to highlight where you worked and/or the positions you have held in a particular field
- You want to highlight career growth in a particular position

The combination résumé. Very simply, this format uses the best components of the functional and chronological styles. The format analyzes your work strengths by area of expertise combined with a chronological listing of work experiences. It can include both chronological and skills sections. The combination résumé is the most flexible and allows for designing a very strong résumé, but it is usually longer and less widely accepted by employers. This format is particularly effective when:

- Each position you have held involves a different job description
- You have held internships or volunteer positions that relate directly to your field of interest

You should *not* consider this format when you do not have a lot of time to create your résumé.

Style

Style is critically important because résumés are typically viewed very quickly. Therefore, your résumé has very little time to make an impression. The following are some style tips that will add to the aesthetic value of your résumé:

- Use conservative fonts; do not use more than two font styles and do not use smaller than 10-point font.
- Be concise! Adhere to a two-page maximum, but one page is even better. If you use more than one page, include your name and "page 2" on the second page.
- Do not crowd too much on a page, make good use of white space, emphasize what is most important, and allow at least a 1-inch margin on all sides.
- Use bold, italics, capitalization, and underlining minimally and consistently to emphasize what is most important.

- Balance material on the page so that it is pleasing to the eye. Put the most important information about one-third from the top, do not hide it at the bottom.
- Use high-quality bond paper in white or off-white (beige or ivory).
- Print on one side of the paper only.
- Be sure the copy has no blurring, stray marks, or faint letters (a laser printer is preferred for clarity and neatness).
- Avoid phony or stilted language, word repetition, unnecessary words or phrases, and the use of any pronouns, particularly "I."
- Avoid the use of acronyms and abbreviations that the reader may not understand.
- Proofread carefully and then proofread again. Use the spell and grammar check tool on your computer.
- Have several people critique your résumé—someone to proofread, someone familiar with the field, and someone unfamiliar with the field.

The Cover Letter

A résumé should always be accompanied by a cover letter. The cover letter will be read before the résumé and, like the résumé, the average time spent reading the letter will be about 20 seconds. Many of the same principles discussed in the section on résumé writing apply to writing the cover letter. It is important to be concise and clear. The letter is a reader's first impression of your writing and organizational skills. The paper used should match your résumé paper; content, formatting, and style all count.

The first paragraph should talk about how you heard about the position and some of your strengths that relate to the job. Do some research on the company and discuss why this company/organization appeals to you. In the second paragraph, briefly describe your qualifications, skills, and accomplishments. Do not just repeat your résumé. This is your chance to point out your outstanding qualities, to direct the reader's attention to any parts of your résumé that are most relevant, to explain any part of your work history that needs clarification, and to show your personality. Your résumé will fill in the details. In the third paragraph, you should relate yourself to the organization: why you would be a good fit and what you could bring to the company. The last paragraph should contain the fact that your résumé is enclosed, a request for an interview appointment, and how and when the employer may easily contact you. Here are some tips for the letter:

- Be sure to personalize your cover letter. Find out the name of the person who will be reviewing your résumé; never use clichés such as "Dear Sir or Madam" or "To Whom It May Concern." If you cannot get a name, use "Dear Internship Director" or "Dear Employer."
- Be specific, clear, and to the point; keep it to one page.
- Proofread the letter very carefully; double and triple check for spelling and grammatical errors.
- Follow standard business letter format.

- Keep copies.
- Do not forget to sign the letter.
- Be yourself.

A skillful, unique cover letter is the best way to demonstrate your intelligence and personality and get you an invitation for an interview.

The Interview

Your cover letter and résumé worked, and you have an appointment for an interview. The interview process can make even the most self-confident person nervous because so much rides on this face-to-face encounter. Even though some nervous energy is positive, too much may be detrimental to your success. The best way to overcome the sense of dread and foreboding is to prepare, prepare, prepare and to look and sound confident during the interview.

The chances are that your interview will last from 15 seconds to 30 minutes. The interviewer will often make his or her decision about you in the first few seconds or minutes of the interview. The other 25 to 29.75 minutes will be a courtesy to you if you have already been screened out. If, however, the results of the first impression are favorable, the interview will last the full half-hour or longer. Achieving this result requires knowing what's important. Employers and graduate schools are looking for some basic qualities: communication skills, appearance, personality, ability to think, energy level, and leadership potential. Be prepared to demonstrate your possession of each of these qualities.

Keep in mind that an interview is a two-way street. Just as the interviewer wants to know if you are right for the position, you want to know if the position is right for you. The interview is your opportunity to find out about the position, the organization, and the culture, and how these might fit into your career goals.

Basics of Interviewing

Some key points to keep in mind on the day of your interview include:

- Be certain of the date, time, and exact place of the interview (including directions and parking).
- Arrive at least 10 to 15 minutes early. Relax, get a drink of water, check your appearance, collect your thoughts, and visualize a positive interview.
- Carry a pen and notepad to make notes of important points. You might also want to jot down the questions you want to ask. Ask permission to take notes.
- Come equipped with your portfolio, extra copies of your résumé, lists of references, and a pen that is readily accessible.
- Wait for the interviewer to offer to shake hands, and use a good, solid grip—neither brute force nor limp.
- Do not smoke or chew gum.
- Wait until the interviewer sits or invites you to sit before doing so.

Basic Preparations for the Interview

Before the day of your interview:

- Research the school/company/organization using the Internet, printed materials, and conversations with faculty, alumni, students, employees, and others.
- Think through your responses to questions according to the type of interview: direct question/answer, indirect ("tell me about yourself?"), or group or board/committee (several interviews and/or several interviewers). Lists of hundreds of typical interview questions are available at the websites listed at the end of the chapter. It is a good idea to prepare answers to some of the most frequently asked questions. Do not memorize the answers, or they will sound too rehearsed.
- Think of questions you want to ask. Your questions will reflect your interest, intelligence, personality, thought processes, and curiosity.
- Assess what you have to offer and be prepared to express that.

The Interview Itself

During the interview you have to communicate your motivation, experience, and skills as well as project your personality. In order to do this:

- Be sincere, courteous, tactful, and enthusiastic.
- Be thorough but concise in your answers.
- Keep the interviewer's attention by being articulate and varying the tone, volume, and tempo of your voice. Speak clearly and audibly.
- Control the content of the interview. Interviewers will ask specific questions. Your responses should directly address the questions and can then smoothly transition to an area or subject that you want to talk more about.
- Presenting your portfolio at the beginning of the interview and asking the interviewer whether he or she would like to look at it now or later, puts you in control from the beginning.
- You may also highlight your answers to questions asked by selecting examples of your work in your portfolio as proof of your experience or skill level.
- Display interest in the interview and treat every question as important.
- Listen carefully to the questions or comments. When they are vague, ask for clarification: "Do I understand your question to be. . . ?"
- Use the "pause-to-think method" (taking your time to organize your thoughts in your mind before responding) when you need to regroup or organize thoughts.
- Avoid negative comments about fellow students, former employers, coworkers, and professors of classes in which your grades were lower.
- Be prepared to respond to questions about your weaknesses as well as your strengths.
- Respond tactfully to questions about your personal life whether or not you understand their relevance to your motivation, qualifications, or goals.
- Be yourself and do not attempt to second-guess what the interviewer would like to hear.

- Do not be intimidated by your competition. Think positively.
- Be prepared for a sophisticated, professional interview technique. If he or she is an experienced interviewer, you will be prepared. If not, you have the advantage.
- Be honest and consistent in your responses.
- Distinguish between questions that call for fact versus those that call for opinion.
- Be confident. Believe in yourself.
- Maintain a comfortable level of eye contact without staring. If you are being interviewed by a group of people, make sure to address all of them with your eyes.
- To break a long silence, say, "May I ask a question about...?" Have some questions ready to ask but avoid questions about salary and benefits at the first interview.
- To redirect the interview to you, ask a question related to something you would be interested in doing (e.g., "Would there be an opportunity during the internship to work on a research project with you or other faculty members, and, if so, when would that be possible?")
- Review your past interviews to improve your techniques for future interviews.
- Encourage yourself.

Closing the Interview

When the interviewer brings the interview to a close, first thank him or her for meeting with you. This should be followed by a question regarding when a decision will be made or what the process is from here.

Tips for Nervousness

It is natural to feel some nervousness before an interview. Some ways to help alleviate this feeling are:

- Get enough sleep before the interview.
- Concentrate on the questions and your responses.
- Take deep breaths and use the pause-to-think method.
- Do not worry about complex questions. If you do not understand a question, do not hesitate to ask for clarification.
- Before and between interviews and in private, practice relaxation techniques by closing your eyes and relaxing one part of your body at a time.

Additional Guidelines

First impressions are important during the interview process. A few additional guidelines for creating a positive first impression are listed below.

- Look neat and clean and dress somewhat conservatively.

    ### Men
    Wear a suit or sport jacket with color-coordinated trousers.
    The color should be neutral—dark-blue, black, or gray is best. Wear a tie.

Shoes should be leather—clean and polished—black is best.

Make sure your nails are trimmed and clean.

Head and facial hair should be neatly trimmed.

Cover any tattoos.

Women

Wear a classic suit or a simple dress with a jacket.

Appropriate colors are navy blue, black, dark green, dark red, burgundy, or gray.

Avoid wearing clothes that are tight, revealing, or trendy.

Fingernails should be trimmed and, if painted, should be in a conservative color.

Hair should be done appropriately—avoid wild hairdos.

Avoid gaudy jewelry and limit pierced jewelry to ears only.
Cover any tattoos.

- Do not wear fragrances, because many people are allergic. Bathing with good-quality bath soap with a mild scent and using an unscented antiperspirant will cover any nervous perspiration.
- Be aware of your posture and avoid distracting "mannerisms," such as foot tapping and touching your hair.
- Remember to turn off your cell phone and/or pager during the interview.
- Write a handwritten thank-you note within 48 hours after each interview. Thank the interviewer for his or her time, again mention your qualifications, and affirm your desire for the position. Do not use email for this note.

Summary

Success in your chosen career in large part depends on knowing yourself. This knowledge allows you to capitalize on your strengths, determine what you want to do and where you want to go, and continuously make improvements in areas that may need strengthening. Beginning to create a student portfolio at the start of your college career is a powerful way to attain this self-knowledge. Toward the end of your college career, turn your student portfolio into a career portfolio. The portfolio creation process requires self-evaluation, reflection, decision making, and goal setting. It has the potential to be a vehicle for career-long professional development and a source of unrivaled personal satisfaction.

A portfolio may also be used as a communication tool to present you and your work to others. While you are a student, your portfolio may be required for evaluative purposes and may actually be graded. When you are a professional, your portfolio is a valuable expansion of your résumé in the interview or job review process. It can be used to generate conversation about your abilities and interests, things you have accomplished, and, perhaps most important, provide actual proof of work you have done (**Figure 4–6**).

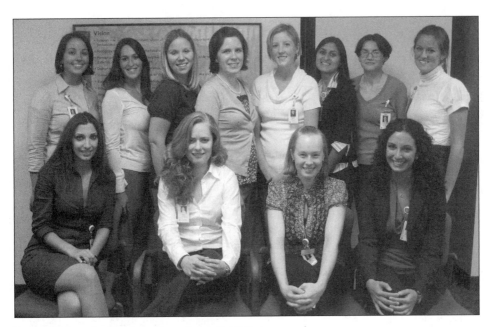

FIGURE 4–6 A graduating class of proud dietetic interns.
Courtesy of Michele Coelho, RD

If your portfolio is a comprehensive view of who you are, your résumé is a snapshot. It is a one- to two-page document that summarizes you and your experiences to attract the attention of potential graduate school directors, employers, colleagues, and others. Because it is the first impression you give a company, presentation and organization of the résumé are critical. Careful attention should be paid to content, format, and style in creating a résumé that will get you an interview.

A cover letter should always accompany a résumé. It is the cover letter that will be read first and very quickly. For these reasons, the cover letter should be clear, concise, personalized, carefully proofread, aesthetically pleasing, and dynamic.

Once an interview is secured, it should be approached with careful preparation and handled professionally. Preparation before the interview includes knowing and understanding your own accomplishments and goals, researching the organization that is interviewing you, thinking of the questions you need to ask, thinking of the answers to questions you may be asked, and being prepared with your portfolio, résumé, and references.

Handling the interview professionally requires that you are well groomed and dressed appropriately, display good manners, and treat everyone with courtesy, stay relaxed and focused, and be yourself.

With a professional portfolio, sharp résumé, and strong interviewing skills, you are on your way to career success in your chosen field of endeavor.

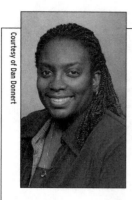

Profile of a Professional

Tandalayo Kidd, PhD, RD, LPN

Assistant Professor and Extension Specialist
Department of Human Nutrition
   Kansas State University
   Manhattan, Kansas

Education:
BS in Nutritional Sciences (Pre-Med), Kansas State University,
   Manhattan, Kansas
MS in Hotel, Restaurant, Institution Management and Dietetics,
   Kansas State University, Manhattan, Kansas
PhD in Human Nutrition, Kansas State University, Manhattan, Kansas

How did you first hear about dietetics and decide to become a Registered Dietitian?
I took a nutrition class and realized how the nutrition profession complemented my nursing background. I did not initially want to become a Registered Dietitian, but as I took more nutrition classes, I began to appreciate the profession and the diverse career paths that dietetics offers.

What was your route to registration?
I completed the Coordinated Program in Dietetics at Kansas State University. My supervised practice experiences were in Housing and Dining Services at K-State and at Salina Regional Health Center in Salina, Kansas.

How are you involved professionally?
I am a member of the Academy of Nutrition and Dietetics, Kansas Dietetic Association, National Organization of Blacks in Dietetics and Nutrition (NOBIDAN), and the American Nurses Organization. I served on the Education and Research Committee for NOBIDAN.

What honors and awards have you received?
I was fortunate to be awarded several scholarships to pursue my education including the Howard Hughes Medical Institute Science Initiative Scholarship and a scholarship from what was then the American Dietetic Association Foundation.

Briefly describe your current position.
I am the nutrition and physical activity specialist for Kansas State Research and Extension. My areas of concentration are obesity, eating disorders, and sports nutrition. My research focuses on young adults and adolescents. As an Extension Specialist, my primary role is to take nutrition-related science information and transform it into usable information for the public. As a researcher, I investigate factors that influence dietary and physical activity behaviors.

What excites you about dietetics and the future of our profession?
The dietetics profession offers a variety of career paths. Human beings are complex; therefore, one career pathway will not satisfy the myriad of needs and desires identified by the majority. I appreciate the diversity from being a clinical dietitian to conducting research to working with the Olympics. Everyone eats; therefore, nutrition is important. I believe the profession will continue to grow because of the emerging science that shows a strong correlation between disease and dietary intake.

How is teamwork important to you in your position?
Teamwork is very important because more things can be accomplished collectively versus individually. For K-State Research & Extension, I work collaboratively with other state specialists and county agents to meet the needs of Kansas residents. In research, I work collaboratively with researchers from other states to meet the needs of a larger audience. Regardless of the setting, each person in a team brings a specific skill set or focus to a project to meet the goals of the project.

What words of wisdom do you have for future dietetics professionals?
Think beyond the traditional clinical dietitian's role. Identify things you are passionate about and then see how the dietetics profession complements that passion. For example, I like being creative, I enjoy working with people, and I want the work that I do to make a difference. Working in Extension with a dietetics and nursing background allows me the opportunity to develop programs and nutrition education materials that can be used to assist many in adopting healthier lifestyle behaviors.

Suggested Activities

1. Ask a classmate or friend to list five adjectives that describe you. Try to use these in writing your personal statement.

2. Print out some of the lists of potential interview questions from the websites listed at the end of this chapter. Think of answers you might give if asked any of these questions.

3. Role play actual interviews with classmates, including direct, indirect, and illegal questions that might be asked. (It is illegal to ask any question that might be discriminatory because of race, religion, sex, age, marital status, or national origin.)

4. Need more help with your résumé? Free templates are available online. Search the Internet to find one that is appropriate for you.

5. Check your interview savvy by taking a quiz at http://career.ucla.edu

6. Want to see a sample of a good résumé? Visit your college placement center and ask to see résumé samples.

7. Either working alone or in teams in class, select a position or specific job (e.g., intern, graduate school candidate, part-time diet office clerk) for which you might apply, and write a list of questions that you might ask during the interview.

8. As you begin to develop your portfolio, give some thought to the following questions:

   - What kind of person do I want to become (desirable characteristics and rejected characteristics)? What can I do to achieve this?
   - What are the characteristics that I want and do not want in my career?
   - What can I do to achieve them?
   - What role do I want in the community and professional organizations?
   - What can I do to achieve this?
   - What kind of family life is important to me?
   - What level and variety of activity do I want?
   - How much effort am I willing to exert to achieve my objectives?

   Summarize the answers to these questions into a list of objectives and action plans.

9. List, in order, five personal characteristics that others seem to appreciate most in you. How did each one develop? How could you use each one to greater advantage? List, in order, five personal characteristics that seem to result in difficulties when dealing with others. How did each one develop? What, if anything, has been or could be done about each one? What other setting might tolerate, if not value, the characteristics most?

10. Identify the major areas of your work or student responsibilities. Rate yourself in each area compared with others in your age and work groups (lowest 25%, middle 50%, next 15%, top 10%). What have you done to improve your performance, and what were the results? What are the biggest obstacles to your improving your work or academic performance? What have you done about each, and what were the results?

Selected Websites

- www.collegegrad.com—Résumé, cover letter, and interviewing information
- http://ehe.osu.edu/career-services—Information on interviewing, résumés, and cover letters
- http://gecd.mit.edu/jobs/find/prepare/resume—Site offers tips on preparing résumés and cover letters

Suggested Resources

Portfolios

Houston CA, Venter-Barkley J. Dietetic student portfolio assessment: it's "elementary" using the moSTEP framework as a model. *DEP Line* 2003;24(Winter):5–11.

Langevin DD. Professional portfolio assessment: a tangible documentation of achievement of the competencies. *DEP Line* 2003;24(Winter):12–13.

Payne-Palacio J. *A Portfolio Primer: An Introduction to Profession Portfolios and the Issues Associated with Their Use*. Malibu, CA: Pepperdine University; 2004.

Quinn JE. Use of authentic assessment through student portfolios. *DEP Line* 2003; 24(Winter):1–9.

Rood R, Martin Mildenhall A. "Portfolio" assignment Utah State University Dietetic Internship. *DEP Line* 2003;24(Winter):4–9.

State of Vermont. Teacher/mentor guide to the Vermont Student Development Portfolio. Available at: http://www.state.vt.us/stw/sdpguide.html. Accessed April 8, 2012.

University of Lethbridge, Canada. A guide to the development of professional portfolios. Available at: http://www.uleth.ca/education/sites/education/files/portfolioguide.pdf. Accessed April 8, 2012.

University of Wisconsin–River Falls. Creating a portfolio. Available at: http://www.uwrf.edu /career/portfolios.htm. Accessed April 8, 2012.

Williams AG, Hall KJ, Shadix K, Stokes DM. *Creating Your Career Portfolio*. Upper Saddle River, NJ: Prentice Hall; 2005.

SWOT Analysis

Personal SWOT Analysis. Available at: http://www.mindtools.com. Accessed April 8, 2012.

SWOT Analysis. Available at: http://www.valuebasedmanagement.net/methods_swot_ analysis.html. Accessed April 8, 2012.

SWOT Template. Available at: http://www.whatmakesagoodleader.com/swot_template.html. Accessed April 8, 2012.

Résumés/Cover Letters

Allen JG. The Resume Makeover, 2nd ed. New York: John Wiley & Sons; 2001.

American Dietetic Association. Resume writing tips for entry-level RDs and DTRs. *J Am Diet Assoc.* 2007;107(4):S10.

American Dietetic Association. Sample resume of someone with management-level experience in the dietetics profession. *J Am Diet Assoc.* 2007;107(4):S8–S9.

American Dietetic Association. Sample resume of student or first-time job seeker in the dietetics profession. *J Am Diet Assoc.* 2007;107(4):S7.

Beatty R. *The Resume Kit.* New York: John Wiley & Sons; 2000.

Block J. *101 More Best Resumes.* New York: McGraw Hill; 1999.

CampusAccess.com. Resume and cover letters. Available at: http://www.campusaccess.com /careers/resumes.html. Accessed April 8, 2012.

CollegeGrad.com. Everything you need to know about cover letters. Available at: http://www .collegegrad.com/coverletters. Accessed April 8, 2012.

CollegeGrad.com. Quickstart resumes. Available at: http://www.collegegrad.com/resumes /quickstart/index.shtml. Accessed April 8, 2012.

Massachusetts Institute of Technology. Effective resume writing/how to get started. Available at: http://web.mit.edu/career/www/workshops/onlineworkshops/resume/index.htm. Accessed April 8, 2012.

Ohio State University. The cover letter. Available at: http://ehe.osu.edu/career-services /downloads/cover-letter.pdf. Accessed April 8, 2012.

Ohio State University. The resume. Available at: http://ehe.osu.edu/career-services/downloads /resume.pdf. Accessed April 8, 2012.

vos Savant M. Ask Marilyn. *Los Angeles Times, Parade Magazine* 2004;January 11:16.

Interviewing

American Dietetic Association. Interviewing tips for entry-level registered dietitians. *J Am Diet Assoc.* 2007;107(4):S13.

CampusAccess.com. Interviews. Available at: http://www.campusaccess.com/careers /interviews.html. Accessed April 8, 2012.

Massachusetts Institute of Technology. Effective interviewing/how to get started. Available at: http://web.mit.edu/career/www/workshops/onlineworkshops/interviewing/index.htm. Accessed April 8, 2012.

Ohio State University. The interview. Available at: http://ehe.osu.edu/cs/careers/interview.php. Accessed April 8, 2012.

Preparing for Practice

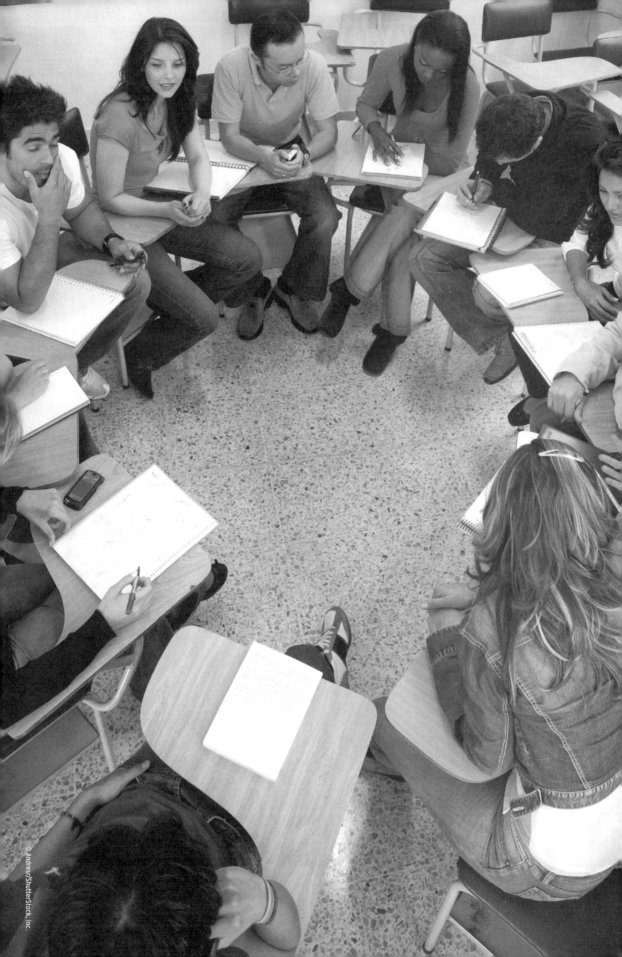

Dietetics Education and Training

Have I Got a Plan for You!

One of the first actions of the fledgling American Dietetic Association (ADA) was the establishment of a teaching section to provide guidance in the education and training of dietitians.[1] From the very earliest days of the profession, academic education has been paired with hands-on, "real-world" experience.[2] The 1927 issue of the *Journal of the American Dietetic Association* published the first "Standardization of Courses for Student Dietitians in Hospitals," as proposed by the section on education of the ADA. Entrance requirements for the hospital-based training program required the dietetic student to be 21 years of age and have a minimum of a bachelor's degree with a major in foods and nutrition from a college or university of "recognized rank."[3]

Many of the subsequent journal articles through the years focused on the hospital portion of the student dietitian's training more than on the academic preparation that preceded the hands-on experience. Early on, the challenge of preparing individuals for the real world of dietetics practice was evident. Mary W. Northrop, a dietitian at Montefiore Hospital in New York City, stated in 1929, "We must take the college girl who comes to us and make her into a professional woman; that six months is too short a time in which to accomplish so complete a metamorphosis is obvious. It seems probable that we shall be forced either to increase the length of our courses or to demand that the colleges send us more mature and competent students."[4]

Times have certainly changed since Ms. Northrop wrote that article! Yes, the dietetics profession is still predominately female, but education programs have advanced beyond "taking the college girl and making her into a professional woman!" Men are joining our profession in increasing numbers; so to the men reading this chapter, please don't despair. Dietetics education programs strive to make professionals of both genders!

The suggested course of study found in the December 1940 issue of the *Journal of the American Dietetic Association* may look vaguely familiar to today's dietetics majors. General chemistry, organic chemistry, and biochemistry were required, as well as human anatomy and physiology, psychology, sociology, economics, educational psychology, food preparation, advanced courses in nutrition, and numerous courses in quantity cookery, organization, and management.[5]

Since 1947, the educational requirements for entry-level dietitians have been revised several times. The last version—"Eligibility Requirements and Education Standards"—was published in 2008. Standards are published individually for each kind of dietetics education program: Didactic Program in Dietetics (DPD), Coordinated Program in Dietetics (CP), International Coordinated Program in Dietetics (ICP), Dietetic Internship (DI), and Dietetic Technician program. The current academic requirements for each program may be found on the Academy of Nutrition and Dietetics website www.eatright.org.[6]

For many years, the only way to become a dietitian was to obtain a BS degree that met the organization's academic requirements, followed by completion of a post-baccalaureate dietetic internship. In 1962, however, the first Coordinated Program in Dietetics was developed, which combined the required internship with the academic program. The student's hands-on experiences were coordinated with what was being discussed in the classroom, with the goal of making the combined learning experience even more meaningful. Through the CP, a student could theoretically fulfill the academic and internship requirements in 4 years rather than 5. Standards for the International Coordinated Program in Dietetics (ICP) were introduced in 2008.

In the early 1970s, the need for dietetic support personnel led to the development of associate degree programs for dietetic technicians. These programs combined a 2-year associate degree with 450 hours of hands-on experience.

The Certified Dietary Manager, Certified Food Protection Professional (CDM, CFPP), a credential awarded by the Association of Nutrition & Foodservice Professionals (ANFP). Individuals with this credential act in a supervisory capacity in food production management and sanitation and, in some practice settings, monitor nutritional status in consultation with a registered dietitian. Find out more information about the CDM, CFPP credential at http://anfponline.org/Training/index.shtml.

The Accreditation Council for Education in Nutrition and Dietetics

The Accreditation Council for Education in Nutrition and Dietetics (ACEND) is recognized as the accrediting agency for associate-degree Dietetic Technician programs, baccalaureate-level DPDs, baccalaureate and graduate-level CPs, and post-baccalaureate DIs. According to the Academy website:

> *ACEND serves the public by establishing and enforcing eligibility requirements and accreditation standards that ensure the quality and continued improvement of nutrition and dietetics education*

*programs that reflect the evolving practice of dietetics. ACEND
defines educational quality as the ability to prepare graduates with
the foundation knowledge, skills and/or competencies for current
dietetics practice and lifelong learning.*[7]

ACEND has a 15-member board.[8] In addition, a group of peer reviewers
with expertise in dietetics education and practice is appointed by ACEND, as
needed, to visit and evaluate programs and make recommendations on accreditation. Currently, 124 of these peer reviewers have been trained to evaluate
and assist dietetics education programs in the accreditation process.[9] ACEND
functions as the governing unit and grants final accreditation awards.

ACEND's Standards and the Accreditation Process

ACEND outlines five standards that must be met by every dietetic education
program:

- **Standards on Program Eligibility for ACEND Accreditation.** These standards relate to program sponsorship, organization, financial resources,
  and leadership. The goal is to make sure the program has a structure in
  place that will ensure success in achieving program excellence.
- **Standards on Program Planning and Outcomes Assessment.** These
  standards are designed to ensure that the dietetic education program
  has a clearly stated mission, goals, and objectives. The program must
  have an assessment process in place with appropriate outcome measures that allows for on-going program improvement and determining
  if the program's goals and objectives have been met.
- **Standards on Curriculum and Student Learning Objectives.** These standards help to make sure the program's curriculum gives students the
  proper foundation in the areas that form the basis of dietetics practice
  (biomedical, nutritional, behavioral, managerial and clinical sciences).
  The content and sequencing of the curriculum and the type of practice
  experiences must be appropriate to prepare graduates for successful
  careers. Methods of promoting student learning and development of
  lifelong learning skills and the assessments to measure these must be
  documented.
- **Standards on Program Staff and Resources.** These standards help to
  ensure that the dietetics program has fair policies and procedures and
  capabilities to attract, develop, and retain well-qualified faculty
  and staff so that the program's goals and objectives can be achieved.
  The program must also demonstrate that it has adequate and appropriate facilities and resources to offer a high quality program.
- **Standards on Students.** These standards help to ensure that the program
  provides adequate resources as well as fair policies and procedures
  to support students and their progression and personal/professional
  development.[6]

Before a dietetic program can begin accepting students, the program's director and faculty members must undertake an in-depth review process known as
a *self-study*. The process for conducting a self-study is outlined in ACEND's
"Candidacy for Accreditation document."[6] The self-study document outlines,

in detail, how the dietetic program meets the ACEND standards. The written self-study document is then forwarded to ACEND and selected peer reviewers.

In previous years, this written self-study was all that was required for certain types of dietetics programs. If peer reviewers deemed that the program's self-study document adequately showed how the program was meeting the standards, the program was "approved" by the accrediting body. However, ACEND now requires that all dietetic education programs be accredited. **Accreditation** means that the program not only writes a self-study document, but the peer reviewers also visit the program to verify that what was written in the self-study document is actually occurring. These site visits are opportunities for the program faculty to interact with the peer reviewers as they work together to ensure that the program's graduates are well prepared and ready for dietetics practice. The site visits also show students, parents, administrators, and others that the dietetic education program meets the high standards set.

A dietetic education program that offers only the coursework necessary to meet the accreditation standards is called a Didactic Program in Dietetics (DPD). A dietetic education program that offers only the supervised practice experiences necessary to meet ACEND standards is called a Dietetic Internship (DI). Coordinated Programs (CPs), International Coordinated Programs (ICPs), and Dietetic Technician programs provide both the academic component and the required supervised practice experience within the degree program. Thus, the self-study document for these programs must outline how both the academic and supervised practice requirements are met for their respective types of programs.

Grievance/Complaint Procedure

If any individual, such as a student, faculty member, dietetics practitioner, or member of the public, has a complaint about an accredited dietetics education program, he or she may submit a complaint or grievance to ACEND. ACEND has established a process for reviewing complaints to fulfill its public responsibility for ensuring the quality and integrity of the educational programs that it accredits. However, ACEND makes it clear that "it will not intervene on behalf of individuals or act as a court of appeal for individuals in matters of admissions, appointment, promotion, or dismissal of faculty or students. It will act only upon a signed allegation that the program may not be in compliance with the accreditation standards or policies." The procedure for complaints against programs can be found on the Academy's website at www.eatright.org.[10]

The Steps to Becoming a Registered Dietitian or Dietetic Technician, Registered

A Registered Dietitian is a food and nutrition expert who has met the minimum academic and professional requirements to qualify for the RD credential. Many RDs deliver medical nutrition therapy in hospitals, HMOs, private practice, or other healthcare facilities. In addition, a large number of RDs work in community and public health settings, in academia, and in research. RDs also work in facets of the food industry, such as school foodservice, college and university foodservice, healthcare foodservice, food manufacturing and sales, corporate wellness programs, and sports nutrition.[11]

A Dietetic Technician, Registered (DTR) is a food and nutrition practitioner who has completed at least a 2-year associate's degree at a U.S. regionally accredited university or college, required coursework, and at least 450 hours of supervised practice accredited by ACEND or at least a bachelor's degree at a U.S. regionally accredited university or college and required coursework for a DPD. A DPD graduate who has had no supervised practice during his or her educational program may want to obtain supervised practice experience to better prepare for the credentialing examination and the job market. In addition, the individual must pass a national DTR examination administered by the Commission on Dietetic Registration (CDR) and complete continuing professional educational requirements to maintain registration. The majority of DTRs work with RDs in a variety of employment settings, including health care (assisting RDs in providing medical nutrition therapy), in hospitals, HMOs, clinics, or other healthcare facilities. In addition, a large number of DTRs work in community and public health settings, such as school or day care centers, correctional facilities, weight management clinics, and WIC programs.[12]

The steps in the preparation for dietetics practice are academic preparation, supervised practice, confirmation of academic preparation by verification from the program director, confirmation of supervised practice by verification from the program director, and credentialing by passing the Registration Examination for Dietetic Technicians or the Registration Examination for Registered Dietitians. These steps apply whether you wish to become a DTR or an RD.

To Become a DTR, You Must...

There are three options by which one may become a DTR:

1. Completion of a 2-year associate degree granted by a U.S. regionally accredited college/university, completion of Dietetic Technician Program requirements in an ACEND-accredited program, a passing score on a national computerized examination administered by the CDR, and completion of continuing professional educational requirements to maintain registration. A specific grade-point average may be required for the student to participate in supervised practice activities. Check with the program director for specific program requirements (**Figure 5–1A**).

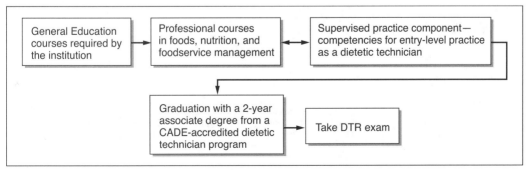

FIGURE 5–1A Dietetic Technician Education Option 1. A specific grade-point average or other criteria may be required for the student to participate in supervised practice activities. Check with the program director for specific program requirements.

2. Completion of a baccalaureate degree granted by a U.S. regionally accredited college/university, or foreign equivalent; completion of an ACEND-accredited DPD, and completion of an ACEND-accredited technician program supervised practice (**Figure 5–1B**).

3. Completion of a baccalaureate degree granted by a U.S. regionally accredited college/university, or foreign equivalent; completion of an ACEND-accredited DPD or CP program; a passing score on a national computerized examination administered by the CDR, and completion of continuing professional educational requirements to maintain registration (**Figure 5–1c**).[13]

To Become an RD, You Must...

1. Complete the minimum of a baccalaureate degree in an accredited DPD or CP that meets ACEND's "Core Knowledge for the RD." Completion of the academic requirements must be verified with a signed Verification Statement from the program director.

2. Complete a minimum of 1,200 hours of supervised practice experience within an accredited CP or accredited DI that meets ACEND's "Core Competencies for the RD." Completion of the supervised practice requirements must be verified with a signed Verification Statement from the program director.

3. Successfully complete the national Registration Examination for Dietitians (**Figures 5–2** and **5–3**).

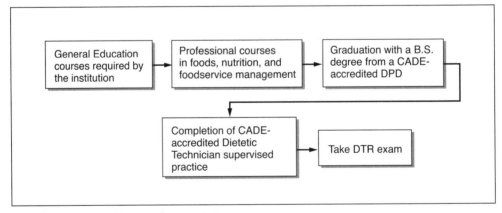

FIGURE 5–1B Dietetic Technician Education Option 2.

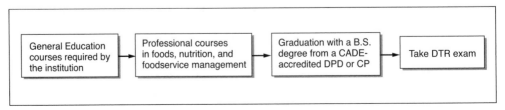

FIGURE 5–1C Dietetic Technician Education Option 3.

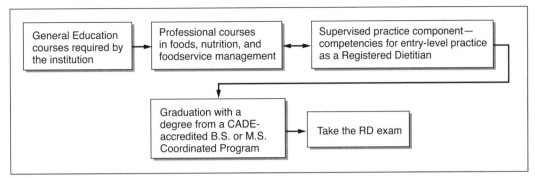

FIGURE 5–2 Coordinated Program in Dietetics (may culminate in a baccalaureate or a master's degree). A separate application process for admission to the supervised practice component of the program is typically required. Every supervised practice program has its own admissions criteria and application process. Check with the program director for further information.

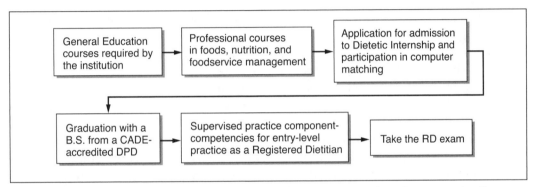

FIGURE 5–3 Didactic Program in Dietetics Plus Dietetic Internship. Every supervised practice program has its own admission criteria and application process. Dietetic internships may have an optional or required graduate education component. Submission of GRE scores and/or acceptance to graduate school may be part of the application process. Check with the program director for further information.

Note: If you already have the minimum of a baccalaureate degree in any area and wish to pursue becoming a Dietetic Technician, Registered or a Registered Dietitian, you must first have your transcripts evaluated to ascertain what additional courses you will need to take to meet the current ACEND knowledge requirements. This evaluation must be completed by the program director at the ACEND-accredited academic program to which you are seeking admission. Earning an additional degree in dietetics may or may not be required, depending on the policies of the institution. Once the appropriate academic requirements have been completed, you may then pursue application to the appropriate supervised practice experience program and finally sit for the credentialing examination.

If You Already Have a Baccalaureate Degree, You Must . . .

If you already have the minimum of a baccalaureate degree in any area and wish to become a DTR or an RD, you must first have your transcripts evaluated to ascertain what additional courses you will need to take to meet the current ACEND "Core Knowledge for the RD." This evaluation must be completed by the program director at the ACEND-accredited academic program to which you are seeking admission. Earning an additional degree in dietetics may or may not be required, depending on the institution's policies. Once the appropriate academic requirements have been completed, you may then pursue application to the appropriate supervised practice experience program and then sit for the credentialing examination.

The Academy website includes additional resources that depict the various education pathways for dietetics students. These can be found on the Academy "Student Center" portion of the Academy of Nutrition and Dietetics website at www.eatright.org.[14]

The Academic Experience

The academic preparation to become a dietitian may be obtained in either an accredited DPD or CP. Dietetic technician students obtain their academic preparation in an accredited Dietetic Technician Program. The dietetics curriculum may be slightly different at different universities, because each school has unique strengths and resources. Graduates of DPDs are eligible to apply for post-baccalaureate supervised practice programs to meet the Academy's requirements. CP graduates meet both the academic and supervised practice requirements in their degree programs and are eligible to sit for the Registration Examination for Dietitians upon completion of their degree (**Figure 5–2**). Likewise, graduates of an accredited Dietetic Technician Program meet both the academic and supervised practice requirements in their associate's degree program and are eligible to sit for the Registration Examination for Dietetic Technicians upon completion of their program.

What knowledge, skills, and abilities are necessary for dietetics professionals to meet the needs of the marketplace in the days ahead? How should dietetics education respond to the Academy's strategic plan and the identified emerging dietetics-related issues of obesity, aging, complementary care, dietary supplements, safety of the food supply, and genetic engineering? Dietetics educators face many challenges in building the best curriculum to answer these and many other questions. Each dietetics education program builds the curriculum to prepare students for the dynamic future of dietetics. Because communication skills are so critical for success in dietetics practice, courses in composition and speech are included. Dietetics practice is grounded in science; thus, courses in biology, anatomy and physiology, microbiology, and chemistry are part of a student's program of study. Having a foundation in these subjects enables students to understand concepts in their professional foods and nutrition courses.

Courses in psychology and sociology help future dietitians understand how people think and act, either individually or in groups. Courses in business, such as economics, marketing, and accounting, prepare students for the managerial and business aspects of dietetics practice, which must be understood no matter what area of dietetics a person might pursue. Because the public eats so many meals away from home in restaurants, fast-food operations, cafeterias, and so on, future dietitians need to understand how food is prepared and served to the public. Basic foods courses help dietetics students learn food science principles and food preparation for the home; however, quantity foods courses prepare students to work with clients in the institutional or commercial foodservice arenas. Courses in normal nutrition, public health nutrition, medical nutrition therapy, and nutritional counseling prepare students for nutritional assessment, diagnosis, and intervention with individuals and groups.

Because the profession of dietetics holds so many options and opportunities, the choice of electives in a student's educational program can build skills in areas that may be useful in the future. Being able to speak another language will be increasingly important as our society becomes more and more diverse. Going beyond the basics of word processing and spreadsheet development to learn more about technology can open doors and enhance the application of technology to dietetics practice. Taking additional courses in business, such as finance, organizational behavior, or entrepreneurship, can prepare students for cutting-edge opportunities. Coursework in gerontology can prepare students to work with the rapidly growing elderly segment of our society. The list of possible elective courses is extensive. The curricula of dietetic education programs will continue to evolve as the profession of dietetics continues to change and grow.

Students who are participating in a coordinated program in dietetics or a Dietetic Technician Program will have courses that have a supervised practice component. A dietetic education program with a supervised practice component (Dietetic Technician Program, CP, or DI) also must include a concentration area as part of the curriculum. The concentration area doesn't mean that the student becomes a specialist in the area, but rather allows the student to gain some additional depth in a particular aspect of dietetics practice. The concentration area(s) is chosen on the basis of the mission, goals, resources, and expected learning outcomes developed by the program.

The Academy website lists 226 ACEND-accredited DPDs. DPDs are available in the District of Columbia, Puerto Rico, and all states. Some states have numerous accredited DPDs: Texas has 16, California has 16, and Illinois has 11. Currently, 53 CPs and 47 Dietetic Technician Programs are accredited by ACEND. The Academy website lists programs by state and distinguishes those programs that offer distance education, those that have course credit transfer agreements, and those that offer graduate degrees.[15] CPs, DIs, and Dietetic Technician Programs—all of which meet ACEND's supervised practice requirement—are discussed in greater detail in the next chapter.

Distance Education in Dietetics

Distance education is defined as "planned learning that normally occurs in a different place from teaching and as a result requires special techniques of course design, special instructional techniques, and special methods of communication by electronic and other technology, as well as special organizational and administrative arrangements."[16] Distance education is a growing phenomenon in education today, and the world of dietetics education is no exception. At present, three DPDs offer the complete baccalaureate degree in dietetics online. Three CPs, 16 DIs, and 3 Dietetic Technician Programs are available in a distance education format.[15] Many programs offer some coursework by distance education. Because of the increasing interest of the public in food and nutrition issues, more and more individuals are interested in the profession of dietetics as a career. Because of the flexibility and asynchronous nature of distance education, this format particularly meets the needs of students who are working in full-time jobs and/or have family responsibilities that may prevent them from taking classes during the day or relocating to a university with a dietetics program.

Many modes of distance education delivery are possible. Although print-based correspondence courses are still available, many universities are using a wide variety of technologies to bring the classroom into the student's home or workplace. Online courses, CD courses, videotaped courses, audio-conferencing, videoconferencing, or combinations of these formats may be used. Some distance programs offer their complete curriculum in a distance format, both general education and professional courses. Other schools may offer degree-completion programs, in which students take the first 2 years of general education courses at a local community college or other institution and then enroll in the distance education program to complete the "professional" foods, nutrition, and foodservice management courses.

Distance education technology may also be used by dietetics programs to offer flexibility in their on-campus courses. Traditional "face-to-face" classes may also use a web support page as a means of posting the course syllabus, maintaining an online grade book, offering a course message board or "chat room" options, and posting other information. On-campus students may use distance technology to interact with off-campus counterparts. Moreover, distance education technology is being used to provide continuing education to credentialed dietetics professionals. Online graduate programs are beginning to appear, and continuing education short courses are increasing. Educational technology is here to stay!

Is distance education right for you? The pros and cons of distance education have been widely discussed. Positive factors include:

- Convenience—the course may be as close as your computer with an Internet connection.
- Flexibility—you can attend class on your schedule because the material is available 24 hours a day, 7 days a week.
- Availability—more and more universities are providing distance education coursework.
- Accessibility—you can work anywhere you have computer access.
- Self-directed—you have more control over the learning environment and can set your own pace or schedule.
- Cost—taking courses online is usually cheaper than incurring moving costs and other expenses involved in relocating to a traditional university setting.

Negative aspects of distance learning include:

- No campus atmosphere—part of the traditional college experience is actually being on campus, soaking up the atmosphere, and experiencing traditional college life.
- Limited social interaction—you do interact with classmates and instructors via email, chat rooms, and discussion groups, but you miss some of the social interaction that is often part of the traditional on-campus experience.
- No face-to-face time with the instructor—the amount of one-on-one interaction you have with the course instructor varies from course to course and university to university. However, if you are the kind of student who likes personal attention from your instructor, distance education may not be for you.

- Making time—if you are a procrastinator or if you need a push to complete your work, you may have a difficult time with the self-discipline necessary to work independently in distance classes.
- Requires new skills and technology—if you are "technophobic" and are uncomfortable with computers and technology, then online education may be a struggle for you, at least in the beginning.
- Expense—you may need specific computer hardware or software to participate in the distance education program, which may lead to additional expense.
- Test taking—you may need to go to a specific location for proctored examinations or to make other special arrangements for taking tests.[17]

When making decisions about a distance education course or program, use the same decision-making steps you would take in deciding about which traditional school to attend:

- Check out the program thoroughly. How long has it been in existence? Is/are the university and program accredited by the appropriate accrediting agencies? How many people are enrolled in the program; how many have graduated? What is the success rate of this program's graduates in obtaining a post-baccalaureate dietetic internship? In passing the RD or DTR exam?
- Talk to other people. Ask if you can interact with current students or graduates of the program. See what they have to say about the quality of the courses and the level of interaction with faculty. What kind of response time did they experience between the time they posed a question and the time they got an answer? What kind of feedback and assistance did they get from faculty?
- Visit by email, phone, or in person, if possible, with the program director. Talk to that person about the program, its philosophy, and its goals. What kinds of resources will be made available to you as a distance education student? As a distance education student, how are you made to feel a part of the university and the program? Do your best to ascertain if you are a good fit for the program.

Distance education is the wave of the future in entry-level education and continuing education. Whether you experience distance education technology in a few courses or whether your whole degree program is obtained in this way, you are probably getting a first taste of the educational delivery system of the future.

Service Learning in Dietetics

Another type of pedagogy that is becoming more and more common in today's dietetics education programs is service learning. Service learning is defined as "a teaching method that combines explicit academic learning objectives with community service."[18] Nothing reinforces abstract, theoretical concepts discussed in class like the opportunity to try out those concepts in a real-life situation benefiting the student's community. Service learning can make textbook theories come alive for students.

According to Chabot and Holben,[19] service learning has numerous advantages for dietetic students. You can acquire both social skills and academic knowledge while enhancing your ability to work with diverse individuals and groups. Assignments have more meaning when they are part of a service learning project rather than a "dry" academic exercise. Participating in service learning can help meet real needs and help you feel more connected to your community. Service learning fosters citizenship, personal development, social responsibility, interpersonal skills, and tolerance. Finally, service learning can provide you with an opportunity for career exploration and can lead to employment opportunities. Chabot and Holben[19] give examples of service learning placements, including working at local soup kitchens and homeless shelters; volunteering with Meals-on-Wheels programs; working with groups such as the American Red Cross, the American Cancer Society, the American Heart Association, and other similar groups; participating with Habitat for Humanity, Big Brothers/Big Sisters, and local hospice organizations. The list goes on and on. Assisting professionals who work in such organizations and seeing what they do and how they do it provides valuable learning experiences for future dietetics professionals.

Verification of Academic Requirements

Upon successful completion of the academic program, the student is issued a Verification Statement. This form is a legal document and should be treated as such. This document, bearing the original signature of the program director, verifies that the student has successfully completed the academic portion of entry-level requirements. Students completing a DPD and a post-baccalaureate supervised practice program will have two Verification Statements; students completing a CP or a Dietetic Technician Program will have only one. These statements must be presented when the student changes from student to active membership in the Academy or when the graduate applies for a license to practice dietetics in a state that has licensure for dietetics professionals.

Building a Career Portfolio

According to Williams and colleagues,[20] a portfolio is "a collection of materials designed to show your work or competencies in a specific area." Many dietetic education programs require each student to compile a portfolio during his or her academic program that showcases the student's skill and abilities. Increasingly, portfolios are developed and accessed online. Examples of materials that may be found in a portfolio include the following:

- A statement of originality (indicating that the contents belong to you and asking people viewing the contents to keep the information confidential)
- A statement of your work philosophy
- Career goals
- A brief biography
- Your résumé

- Skill areas, including work samples, letters of recommendation, and skill sets (checklists of critical skills related to the area)
- Works in progress
- Certifications, diplomas, degrees, scholarships, and awards
- Professional memberships/affiliations and certifications
- Academic plan of study
- Supervised practice plans
- Publications
- Faculty and employer biographies
- References

Building and maintaining a career portfolio is an ongoing process. As you move through your schooling and supervised practice experiences, you will continually be adding new material to your portfolio and removing material that may no longer be relevant. As you enter dietetics as a practicing professional, you will create and maintain your career portfolio as part of the CDR credentialing process. Chapter 7 in this text provides more detailed information about the professional development portfolio. Because the portfolio process will be an ongoing part of your life as a dietetics professional, it makes sense for you to start learning about portfolios and building your own now as a student (see also Chapter 4).

Graduate Education

Graduate education has long been valued among dietetics professionals. The Academy of Nutrition and Dietetics's "2011 Dietetics Compensation and Benefits Survey" revealed that 45% of all RDs hold a master's degree, indicating that members of the profession value advanced education. The report noted, "Education beyond the bachelor's degree is clearly associated with wage gains." The report also revealed that 49% of dietetics professionals receive assistance with college tuition as a job benefit.[21]

You might think that the decision of whether to attend graduate school is something far in the future. However, students should keep the possibility in mind even as they are pursuing their undergraduate education. If you think you might like to pursue a master's or doctoral degree someday, remember that academic performance at the undergraduate level is a major criterion for admission to graduate school. Typically, a 3.0 GPA at the undergraduate level is required for a person to be admitted to a graduate program. The applicant may also be required to take a graduate school admissions test, such as the Graduate Records Examination (GRE) or the Graduate Management Admissions Test (GMAT). A review of the applicant's undergraduate GPA, performance on a standardized admissions test, letters of recommendation from professors and/or employers, and a clear and concise statement of goals for graduate study often make up the graduate school admission process.

There are various opinions about whether a student should go straight from an undergraduate program directly into a graduate program or whether the student should work a few years before pursuing graduate study. The graduate school experience is different from the undergraduate program.

Graduate classes are often smaller than undergraduate ones, and classes tend to be more "discussion driven." A student coming straight from his or her baccalaureate program into a graduate program without having much "real-world" experience may find him- or herself somewhat at a loss to contribute to class discussions in the same way as others who have had more work experience in the field. Work experience also allows an individual to hone his or her interests and may be the source of questions that might be answered in a master's thesis or doctoral dissertation!

However, a growing number of post-baccalaureate dietetic internships offer the new graduate the opportunity to pursue a master's degree concurrently with obtaining the required DI experience. Many students find this opportunity exciting, and see the master's degree/internship combination as a chance to further their education in a more in-depth and focused way while meeting the dietetics supervised practice requirements.

Master's degrees may be earned in any number of areas, including the following:

MPH—Master of Public Health

MBA—Master of Business Administration

MS—Master of Science (in a variety of subjects)

MEd—Master of Education

Most master's degree programs require 30–36 credit hours beyond the baccalaureate degree. A master's program may be research oriented, with the student completing both coursework and a research project. The student writes a thesis that incorporates a review of pertinent literature; a description of the research idea/problem, methodology, and data analysis; a description of the findings; conclusions drawn; and recommendations for future research. A master's program may also be non-thesis, meaning that instead of doing a research project the student takes additional coursework. At the conclusion of the program of study, students may be asked to pass a comprehensive written and oral examination over their academic program of study.

Graduate study at the doctoral level also may be completed in a variety of disciplines:

PhD—Doctor of Philosophy (in a wide variety of disciplines)

EdD—Doctor of Education

DSc—Doctor of Science

DBA—Doctor of Business Administration

JD—Doctor of Jurisprudence or Doctor of Law

MD—Doctor of Medicine

Most doctoral programs are considered approximately 90 credit hours of study beyond the baccalaureate degree, about 30 credits hours of which are research. Doctoral degrees involve advanced coursework, completion of a major research endeavor, and the writing and defense of a dissertation. Individuals who complete doctoral degrees often teach in colleges and universities, work as researchers in higher education or in industry, or become chief executive officers of organizations.

The benefits of advanced study are both tangible and intangible. Many people pursue advanced study because of their intrinsic drive to learn and grow. Having an advanced degree may enhance a person's status and enable the person to earn a higher salary or be promoted to new levels of responsibility and authority. Graduate education should also help the individual to understand the research process and to develop teamwork, critical thinking, problem solving, communication, and other skills that can make him or her more marketable and successful in his or her professional endeavors. The Academy website (www.eatright.org) has a list of graduate programs in areas that may be of interest to dietetics professionals.[22]

Summary

Preparation for entry into the profession of dietetics encompasses both prescribed academic preparation and supervised hands-on experience. Both of these components are carefully structured and monitored by the Academy through its Accreditation Council for Education in Nutrition and Dietetics. Ongoing practice audits form the basis for the "Core Knowledge" and "Core Competency" statements used to guide the development of both academic curricula and supervised practice experiences. A complete listing of all accredited dietetic education programs of every type can be found on the Academy website, www.eatright.org.[23]

The challenge facing the Academy and dietetic educators is to keep educational preparation on the cutting edge of professional practice, ensuring that current students will be prepared for the exciting future that awaits them as dietetic technicians and registered dietitians. The most important focus must be on the development of critical-thinking and problem-solving skills, so that future dietitians know how to think, rather than what to think. Future dietitians must be prepared to take responsibility for their own continued professional development, because information about food and nutrition issues is expanding at an exponential rate. By learning how to learn, the dietitian student will be ready for an exciting future in dietetics.

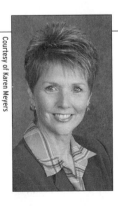

Courtesy of Karen Meyers

Profile of a Professional

Karen Meyers, MS, RD, LD

Owner, NutriFit of Oklahoma
Edmond, Oklahoma

Education:
BS, Nutrition, Dietetics and Food Management, University of
    Central Oklahoma
MS, Nutrition and Food Management, University of Central
    Oklahoma
Purdue University, West Lafayette, Indiana

How did you first learn about dietetics as a profession?
I have a long family history of type 2 diabetes and saw what a difference good nutrition could make in a person's life. Good nutrition has always been a passion of mine, so when I decided to go back to school at the age of 35, I knew it was something I wanted to pursue.

What was your route to registration as a dietitian?

I completed a dietetic internship concurrently with completing a master's degree in Nutrition and Food Management at the University of Central Oklahoma.

Describe your career path thus far.

After completing my internship and passing the RD exam in 1996, I was a clinical dietitian in a hospital and a senior clinic. I also taught as adjunct faculty at the University of Central Oklahoma. In 2000, I became the Dietetic Internship Director and served in that capacity until 2006. In 2006, I began a private practice after becoming a Certified Wellcoach/Health Coach and Certified Personal Trainer through the American Council on Exercise. I currently do some consulting, personal training, and nutrition coaching.

What are some examples of your professional involvement?

2000—Oklahoma Dietetic Association Medical Nutrition Therapy Manual Co-Chairman

2003—Oklahoma City District Dietetic Association Legislative Committee Chairman

2005—American Dietetic Association Leadership Institute Participant

2005—President of the Oklahoma Dietetic Association

2006—American Dietetic Association Affiliates Future Task Force

Have you received honors or awards?

2001—Oklahoma Dietetic Association Outstanding Dietetics Educator Award

2002—Emerging Leader in Dietetics Award

2003—Oklahoma City District Dietetic Association Distinguished Dietitian

How is teamwork important to you in your position?

I realized early in my career that teamwork is very important. In the clinical setting, no one person is able to solve a patient's problem. In education, teamwork means the difference between a student achieving his or her dream or not. In private practice, there are still opportunities for teamwork. I consider each of my clients a very important member of the team.

What words of wisdom do you have for future dietetics professionals?

Think beyond what you think you are capable of! If you need help, find a mentor or coach to get you past any obstacles you might come upon. There are so many opportunities within your reach! Nutrition is an exciting and dynamic field and one in which you are limited only by your imagination!

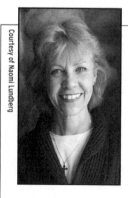

Courtesy of Naomi Lundberg

Profile of a Professional

Naomi R. Lundberg, DTR

Wellness Manager
Valley Natural Foods
Burnsville, Minnesota,

Education:
BS in Health and Biology, minor in Recreation, Bemidji State University, Bemidji, Minnesota
AAS in Dietetic Technology, Normandale Community College, Bloomington, Minnesota

How did you first hear about dietetics and decide to become a Dietetic Technician, Registered?

I have been interested in nutrition and the health field since high school, but I didn't decide to be a dietetic technician until 1998. I was reading a publication from a local community college where a recent graduate of their dietetic technician program was interviewed. It sounded like something I'd like to do.

Describe the supervised practice experiences during your Dietetic Technician program.

I had the opportunity to gain experience in a variety of settings. At the Wilder Community Center, I wrote articles for the community newsletter, developed and taught a class on healthy eating for preschool children, and did visits to licensed day care providers, checking on the nutritional adequacy of their menus. I also had a rotation at the Minnesota Masonic Home where I participated in clinical responsibilities in their assisted-living and skilled-care units. I also worked in food preparation activities, such as doing recipe modifications and learning about modified diets. Finally, I had experiences at Hennepin County Medical Center, where I had clinical experience in cardiac and critical care units doing nutrition assessment and patient education.

Are you involved in professional activities?

I have been a member of the Academy of Nutrition and Dietetics since my graduation in 2001 and active in my home state's association as a member of the silent auction committee, as well as a speaker at the Minnesota Dietetic Association's annual meeting in Rochester, Minnesota. I served for 3 years as a board member on Normandale Community College's dietetics committee and have been a guest speaker for the Minnesota Day Care Providers at their annual meeting in St. Paul.

Have you received recognition for your work?

I write a column in a bimonthly magazine published by Valley Natural Foods in Burnsville, Minnesota. This magazine recently received a national award for excellence for a publication of its size. Also, I have been privileged to have been nominated by my peers for the Outstanding Dietetic Technician, Registered of MN award in both 2009 and 2010.

Describe your career path in dietetics.

After graduation, I worked for 4 years in public health with the Women, Infants, and Children (WIC) program. I am presently employed by Valley Natural Foods as Wellness Manager. My position involves providing education and information on supplements and natural beauty care products. I also have the opportunity to explain the importance of a healthy diet, good nutrition habits, and exercise for the good health of our customers.

What excites you about dietetics and the future of our profession?

The future for dietetics professions remains bright. Now, more people than ever are concerned about what they eat and how to avoid nutritional problems or get help with problems such as obesity and diabetes. Food allergies and intolerances are on the rise, with the need for specialized diets, and baby boomers want to maintain good health to remain active and healthy in their senior years.

How is teamwork important to you in your practice?

Working with a team is a great way to brainstorm solutions and get things done quickly and efficiently. In my job, I am involved with a team to form committees for events, public speaking, and community service. We work together, each with our own expertise and knowledge. It is very effective. Teamwork also involves networking with others, which is always a good thing!

What words of wisdom do you have for future dietetics professionals?

Believe in yourself. Don't settle for "second best." Market yourself by showing your employer that "something extra" that only you can bring to the workplace. Look beyond the traditional path and create a niche!

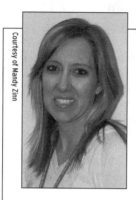

Courtesy of Mandy Zinn

Profile of a Professional

Mandy R. Zinn, CDM, CFPP

Director of Food Service, USD 373
Newton, Kansas

Education:
Dietary Manager course—Wichita Area Technical School, Wichita, Kansas

How did you first hear about dietetics and decide to become a Certified Dietary Manager, Certified Food Protection Professional?
I worked as a dietary aide in a long-term care facility in high school and then moved up to a cook position when I turned 19. The facility I worked at offered to sponsor me to take the dietary management course. I worked full time as a morning cook and went to school in the evenings. I remember a member of the Kansas Dietary Managers Association coming to my class one evening and speaking about becoming a Certified Dietary Manager after my course was completed. She also stressed becoming a member of the Association of Food and Nutrition Professionals (formerly the Dietary Managers Association).

Describe the supervised practice experiences during your technician program.
I worked with an excellent Registered Dietitian at the Bethesda Home, a long-term care facility, in Goessel, Kansas.

Are you involved in professional activities?
I have been a member of the Kansas Association of Nutrition & Foodservice Professionals (formerly the Kansas Dietary Managers Association) for 6 years. Right after becoming a member, I served on one of the association's committees, then became the treasurer for my district association, a position I held for 3 years. I am currently president of the Kansas Association of Nutrition & Foodservice Professionals.

Describe your career path in dietetics.
After working in one long-term care facility as a dietary aide and cook while completing my dietary manager training, I then became the manager of a small assisted-living facility. After a year in that position, I moved to the long-term care area and became the Director of Food Service, a position I held for 6 years. Currently, I am the Director of Food Service for USD 373 school district in Newton, Kansas, where I have been for 15 months.

What excites you about dietetics and the future of our profession?
I love to teach people about nutrition and also working with recipes and menus. There will always be a need for Certified Dietary Managers! We keep up with meal regulations/guidelines, training staff, sanitation, and manage culture change in assisted-living facilities and long-term care. Now I am working with the Healthy Eating in Schools initiative for students. Food and nutrition will always be changing and makes this an exciting area in which to work.

How is teamwork important to you in your practice?
Teamwork is important to me because there are so many areas in my foodservice operation that it takes everyone working together to accomplish our goals every day.

One of our team projects is the Summer Food and Activity Program here in our community. I work with teachers and local community centers to provide free meals and activities for the children of our town in the summer. I plan menus and complete the required paperwork, my staff makes the meals, the teachers plan the activities, and the community center helps with gathering volunteers, advertising, and so on. It's a total team effort.

My school district team has a great relationship with the parents of our students, with the faculty, with other staff, and with the community. We are known for doing a good job of providing meals to the students, catering dinners, preparing and delivering treats for classrooms, providing nutrition education, food for community events, and last, but not least, for having a good time at work. We love to laugh and celebrate every chance we get!

What words of wisdom do you have for future dietetics professionals?
Keep an open mind and step out of the box. We are in a world of change; food and people are ever-changing, so be ready for any challenge that may come at you. I believe being a "great leader" is better than being a "boss." Have a good attitude and you'll go far. Teach your staff good customer service, for it can break or make your dining experience!

Suggested Activities

1. Find out about the history of your dietetics program. When did the program begin? How many people have graduated from your program? What are some of those graduates doing now?

2. Interview a dietitian in your area. Ask the dietitian the following questions:

    a. How did you learn about the profession of dietetics?

    b. What kind of dietetics education program did you go through?

    c. What was your first dietetics position?

    d. What other dietetics positions have you held?

    e. Describe your current job and its responsibilities.

    f. What skills do you believe are necessary for successful dietetics practice?

    g. What do you like best about being a dietitian or dietetic technician?

3. Access the listing of dietetic education programs on the Academy website (www.eatright.org). Are there other dietetics education programs in your state? In a neighboring state? If so, where are they? What kinds of programs are offered? Contact some of the students in these programs and network with them!

4. Select two dietetics programs other than your own. Go to the websites of each program and read about them. Compare the curriculum and experiences of each program with the program in which you are enrolled. What are the commonalities? What are the differences?

5. Review the "Core Knowledge" and "Core Competency" statements for the type of dietetic education program in which you are enrolled. This listing may be found on the Academy website (www.eatright.org). Compare these requirements with your dietetics curriculum to see how your curriculum helps prepare you to meet these requirements.

6. Compare the "Core Knowledge" and "Core Competency" statements for dietetic technicians and registered dietitians. Explain how the education and training for DTRs complement the training of the RD and enable the two professionals to work together in a supportive relationship.

7. Check out dietetics programs that have a distance education option. These may be found on the Academy website (www.eatright.org) under the listing of all accredited programs. How do these programs work? What are the pros and cons of this educational approach? Contact a distance dietetics program and interview one of their students to learn more about the experience.

Selected Websites

- www.eatright.org/BecomeanRDorDTR/content.aspx?id=8146&terms =advanced+degrees—a search engine at the Academy Student Center for advanced degrees
- www.eatright.org/BecomeanRDorDTR/content.aspx?id=8092— Getting started at the Academy student center.
- www.eatright.org/ACEND/content.aspx?id=7877—area of the ACEND website to learn more about the accreditation process and standards for the various types of dietetic education programs.
- www.eatright.org/BecomeanRDorDTR/content.aspx?id=8156—this site contains a listing of all ACEND-accredited dietetic education programs.
- www.eatright.org/ACEND/content.aspx?id=7975—visit this site to learn about the procedures for complaints against an accredited program.

References

1. Cassell J. *Carry the Flame: The History of the American Dietetic Association.* Chicago: The American Dietetic Association; 1990.
2. Otis FA. A combination theory and practice course for student dietitians. *J Am Diet Assoc.* 1925;3:138–140.
3. Section on Education of the American Dietetic Association. Standardization of courses for student dietitians in hospitals. *J Am Diet Assoc.* 1926;12:171–176.
4. Northrop MW. The training of student dietitians. *J Am Diet Assoc.* 1929;5:208–211.
5. Professional Education Section. Chairman's Summary. *J Am Diet Assoc.* 1940;16:1016–1018.
6. American Dietetic Association. Commission on Accreditation for Dietetics Education: 2008 Eligibility Requirements and Accreditation Standards. Available at: http://www .eatright.org/uploadedFiles/CADE/Accreditation/DPD_2008_ERAS_v0-1_2009-07-18_1200.pdf. Accessed January 21, 2010.
7. Academy of Nutrition and Dietetics. ACEND Mission. Available at: http://www.eatright .org/ACEND/content.aspx?id=4294967419. Accessed May 5, 2012.
8. Academy of Nutrition and Dietetics. ACEND Board Members. Available at: http://www .eatright.org/ACEND/content.aspx?id=37. Accessed May 5, 2012.
9. Academy of Nutrition and Dietetics. ACEND Peer Program Reviewers. Available at: http://www.eatright.org/ACEND/content.aspx?id=4294967420. Accessed May 5, 2012.

10. Academy of Nutrition and Dietetics. Procedure for Complaints Against Accredited Programs. Available at: http://www.eatright.org/ACEND/content.aspx?id=7975. Accessed May 5, 2012.

11. Academy of Nutrition and Dietetics. What Is a Registered Dietitian? Available at: http://www.eatright.org/BecomeanRDorDTR/content.aspx?id=8142. Accessed May 5, 2012.

12. Academy of Nutrition and Dietetics. What Is a Dietetic Technician, Registered? Available at: http://www.eatright.org/BecomeanRDorDTR/content.aspx?id=8142. Accessed May 5, 2012.

13. Academy of Nutrition and Dietetics. Education and Professional Requirements for Dietetic Technicians. Available at: http://www.eatright.org/ACEND/content.aspx?id=7981. Accessed May 5, 2012.

14. Academy of Nutrition and Dietetics. Getting Started. Available at: http://www.eatright.org/BecomeanRDorDTR/content.aspx?id=8092. Accessed May 5, 2012.

15. Academy of Nutrition and Dietetics. Accredited Education Programs. Available at: http://www.eatright.org/BecomeanRDorDTR/content.aspx?id=8156. Accessed May 5, 2012.

16. Moore M, Kearsley G. *Distance Education: A Systems View*. Belmont, CA: Wadsworth, 1996:2.

17. Hansen RS. Distance learning pros and cons. Available at: http://www.quintcareers.com/distance_learning_pros-cons.html. Accessed January 23, 2010.

18. Seifer S, Connors K. Improved student learning and community health: the CCPH faculty service learning institute. *Acad Med*. 2000:75;533–534.

19. Chabot JM, Holben DH. Integrating service-learning into dietetics and nutrition education. *Topics Clin Nutr*. 2003:18(3);177–184.

20. Williams AG, Hall KJ, Shadix K, Stokes DM. *Creating Your Career Portfolio: At-a-Glance Guide for Dietitians*. Upper Saddle River, NJ: Prentice-Hall, 2005.

21. Ward, B. Compensation & benefits survey 2009: Despite overall downturn in economy, RD and DTR salaries rise. *J Am Diet Assoc*. 2010:110;25–36.

22. Academy of Nutrition and Dietetics. Advanced Degrees. Available at: http://www.eatright.org/BecomeandRDorDTR/content.aspx?id=8146. Accessed May 5, 2012.

23. Academy of Nutrition and Dietetics. Accredited Dietetic Education Programs. Available at: http://www.eatright.org/ACEND/content.aspx?id=73. Accessed May 5, 2012.

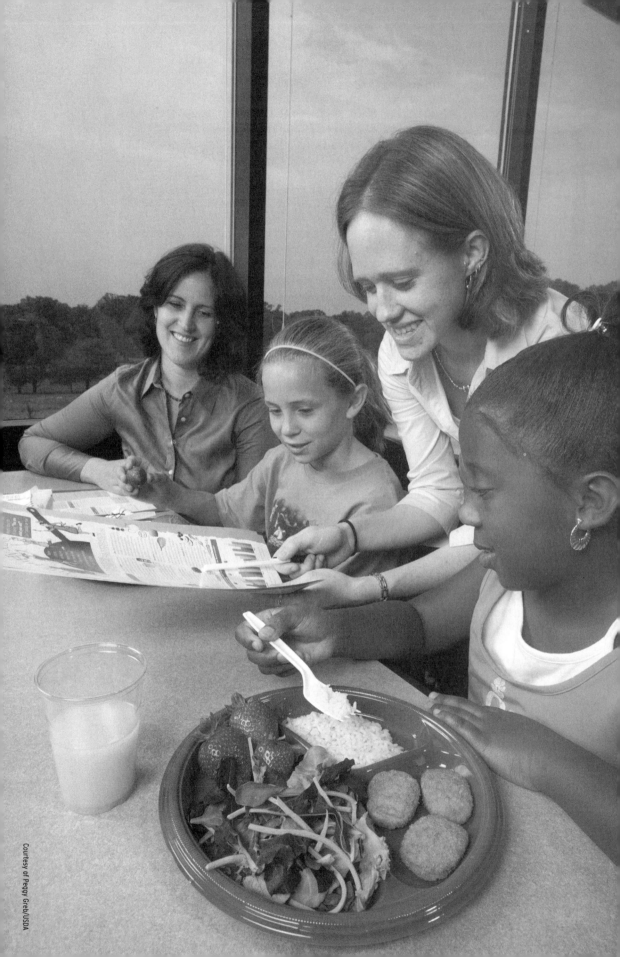

The Supervised Practice Experience

Trying Your Wings

For students wishing to become credentialed dietetics professionals, nothing is more nerve-wracking or more exciting than the process of applying for and being admitted to the supervised practice experience. Students in Dietetic Technician programs participate in a 450-hour supervised practice experience; those pursuing the RD credential must successfully complete 1,200 hours. This chapter discusses the supervised practice experience and how one prepares for, applies for, and gets the most out of this critical step on the path to the dietetics profession.

Supervised practice is the critical time when you have the opportunity to try out the application of theory in the "real world." It is the time when you really see what dietetics professionals do in a variety of work settings, how they spend their time, the decisions they make, the challenges they face, the joys and trials of the job, and the "politics" of the workplace. The dietetics professionals who act as preceptors will become some of the most instrumental people in your professional development. Most of these individuals are not paid to work with students or interns; they do it out of the goodness of their hearts and their desire to help the next generation of food and nutrition professionals. In other words, they are often the "unsung heroes" in the story of dietetics education and training. Whether your supervised practice takes place in one facility or in multiple sites, an incredible amount of planning and coordination has taken place "behind the scenes" to make this learning experience the best possible.

Competencies for the Supervised Practice Component

Just as the Accreditation Council for Education in Nutrition and Dietetics (ACEND) has outlined specific "Core Knowledge" for the academic part of your dietetics education, there are also specific "Core Competencies" for the supervised practice component of both dietetic technician and dietitian education programs.[1,2] As you read through the "Core Competencies," you will see that performance-based and action verbs are used to demonstrate that these are hands-on skills to be developed, readying you for practice in the "real world."

Just as with the didactic portion of dietetics education, the supervised practice competencies have been developed from practice audits and research with practicing dietetics professionals who understand what an entry-level professional should be able to do when arriving on his/her first job. The supervised practice experience is exactly what the name implies. It is a time when you, as a student or intern, can "practice" the competencies expected of a professional while under "supervision." You can hone your skills and get a feel for what the day-to-day activities are like for a dietitian or dietetic technician in a relatively low-risk environment.

Although ACEND dictates that a minimum number of hours must be included in supervised practice, the division of these hours among the different competencies to be achieved is not mandated. Each dietetics program looks at its goals, desired outcomes, and resources and decides how to divide the hours. In other words, to meet the 450- or 1,200-hour requirement, the program does not have to provide one-third of the hours in community nutrition, one-third in foodservice management, and one-third in clinical nutrition. As long as the program can demonstrate by outcome assessment that its graduates are meeting the core competencies, the faculty can design the program to take the best advantage of its resources and meet the specific needs of its constituencies.

When Does Supervised Practice Occur?

Supervised practice programs for dietetic technicians must be a minimum of 450 hours. Supervised practice programs for dietitians must be a minimum of 1,200 hours. The program may opt to include more hours of training if needed to achieve the program goals. This training occurs at different points, depending on the type of program in which the student is enrolled. Some students graduate from a Didactic Program in Dietetics (DPD) and then are admitted to a post-baccalaureate Dietetic Internship (DI). DIs vary in length. Some are as brief and intense as 6 months, during which interns work 40–50 hours per week hours per week to complete the requirements. Others may last 1 or 2 years, especially if graduate coursework or a master's degree is combined with the supervised practice program.

Students in Coordinated Programs in Dietetics (CPs and ICPs) are involved in supervised practice concurrently with their didactic coursework. Some programs may start the supervised practice experience during the junior year and extend the acquisition of the 1,200 hours over three or four semesters. The Academy website also lists 22 CPs/ICPs that provide the opportunity for students to combine graduate coursework with supervised practice, culminating in a master's degree.[3] Likewise, Dietetic Technician programs also have the 450 hours of supervised practice interspersed and sequenced with the didactic coursework.

Making the Decision: Coordinated Program Versus Dietetic Internship

There are 53 CPs in dietetics and 248 dietetic internships in the United States.[3] As previously discussed, CPs combine the supervised practice experience with the academic degree program. These programs were initially designed to speed up the preparation of dietitians by combining the hands-on experience with the degree program and eliminating the post-baccalaureate internship requirement. This means that students in these programs could conceivably be RD-eligible in a shorter period of time.

As with any decision, there are pros and cons to be considered. Students should consider numerous factors before deciding which route to take. Just living close to a particular program doesn't mean that it is the best program for you. Programs have strengths and weaknesses, advantages and limitations, and a culture or "personality"—just like individuals. Wise students do their homework ahead of time by visiting program websites; actually visiting the program to talk to faculty and students, if possible; and checking out program statistics before making the all-important decision to apply for admission.

CPs often draw their students from a more regional area, whereas DIs may attract students from across the country. Because supervised practice hours are built into the program, CPs are intense and allow for few unrestricted electives. However, CP graduates are immediately eligible to sit for the RD exam, and thus enter practice sooner than their internship-bound classmates. Students who decide to enroll in a didactic program followed by an internship may have more unrestricted electives; thus, it may be easier for them to gain a minor or second major during their undergraduate program. Interns may be able to combine graduate coursework or a full master's degree program along with their internship. Although there are some master's-level CPs, most CPs tend to culminate in a baccalaureate degree. Obviously, each type of program has its pros and cons, and only you can decide which type of program is best for you.

Another great resource for decision making is the *Applicant Guide to Supervised Practice*, a publication of the Nutrition and Dietetic Educators and Preceptors (NDEP) Dietetic Practice Group (DPG) of the Academy. This publication is updated annually and may be purchased from the NDEP DPG.[4] Your program director also may have a copy on reserve in his or her office or in your school library. Not all supervised practice programs may choose to include their information in this publication. However, the document contains a wealth of information about supervised practice programs that choose to submit information. Information includes the cost of the program, entrance requirements, factors considered in evaluating applications, kinds of facilities used for experiences, typical numbers of students applying, acceptance rates, and other information that is difficult to find from traditional resources.

Every year, many DIs host open houses so that prospective applicants can learn more about the various programs available. Keep in touch with your didactic program director, because he or she may be notified about these open houses. Also, during student activities at the annual Food and Nutrition Conference and Exhibition (FNCE) of the Academy, DIs often set up displays and information tables about their programs.

A good way to acquire information about supervised practice is to visit the Student Center website, an area on the public Academy website (www .eatright.org) that is chock-full of great information for students. The Members Only section of the Academy website offers additional information for Academy student members about improving one's chances of getting an internship placement, student tips for success in supervised practice, and information about the availability of DIs.[5]

Other sources for information and guidance about the DI application process are the websites set up by DIs themselves. Because being selected for a DI is increasingly competitive, students can benefit from these informative sites and gain insight into what each program may be looking for in applicants.

Distance Internships

A relatively new phenomenon in the world of supervised practice is the "distance internship." As distance education didactic programs in dietetics have grown, the idea of distance internships has also become a reality. The Academy website currently lists 16 internships that offer distance education options.[6] These programs work with each intern to select facilities in the location where the intern lives and to design a personal internship experience for that student. Every program has its own policies and procedures. If this sort of program sounds as if it may meet your needs, visit the websites of these programs and see whether such a program may be right for you.

Individualized Supervised Practice Pathways (ISPPs)

Individualized supervised practice pathways or ISPPs were introduced in September 2011 by the Academy. These programs provide students the opportunity to gain the required knowledge and skills for dietetics practice by working under the guidance of individual practitioners with direction from an ACEND-accredited dietetics program. Individuals who can take advantage of an ISPP are limited to 1) graduates who did not match to a dietetic internship but who hold a DPD verification statement, 2) individuals who hold a doctoral degree, or 3) overseas dietitians who wish to become credentialed to practice in the United States. ACEND-accredited programs sponsoring an ISPP may have different eligibility requirements and options, so if you believe you qualify for this supervised practice route, you must investigate the options provided by sponsoring programs. Check the ISPP site on the Academy website for more detailed information at: http://www.eatright.org /ACEND/content.aspx?id=6442465002.[7]

Applying for the Supervised Practice Experience

The supervised practice experience application process can be broken down into the following steps.

Step 1: Gain Dietetics-Related Work Experience

Start early by gaining dietetics-related work experience. This may be paid experience or volunteer experience. Gain experience in as many different areas of dietetics practice as you can. You will learn much about the breadth and depth of the profession of dietetics, which will better prepare you to take advantage of your supervised practice experiences. Some supervised practice programs may require you to have a certain number of hours of work experience before you apply to the program. Such work experience is highly recommended for all students and will only strengthen your application. You can obtain dietetics-related work experience in a number of ways:

- Volunteer with a WIC program.
- Deliver Meals-on-Wheels to the elderly.
- Work at a health fair with a dietetics professional.
- Work as a diet aide in a hospital or long-term care facility.
- Shadow dietitians in various areas of dietetics practice, and observe what they do and how they do it.
- Gain work experience in foodservice operations in food preparation and service. Look for part-time jobs in hospital or nursing home kitchens, restaurants, summer camps, or other foodservice operations.
- Look for shadowing or volunteer opportunities with dietetics professionals who work in nontraditional areas of practice, such as those working with the media or on the Internet; RDs in private practice consulting, sales, and marketing; and other entrepreneurs.

Step 2: Investigate the Available Supervised Practice Programs

Investigate the wide array of available supervised practice programs. The Academy website (www.eatright.org) has a complete list of CPs, DIs, and Dietetic Technician programs; this includes a brief description of the program, the program director's name, the website for the program, and contact information for the program director.[8]

Visit the websites of the various programs, and, if you need further information, contact the program director. Take advantage of any open house opportunities that the program may provide or call and ask if you can make special arrangements to visit the program. Read the program description carefully to determine whether the focus of the program is in line with your interests.

Step 3: Narrow Your Choices

Narrow your choices and decide on the programs to which you wish to apply. Remember that putting together a "letter-perfect" application takes considerable time and effort, so be selective in your efforts. Also, do not "put all your eggs in one basket." Applying to only one program can be risky, because competition is strong for supervised practice placements. Applying to only one program and not being selected can be a devastating experience. Carefully think through your top five to eight choices. Think long term. Do not pick a supervised practice program because it is convenient or because it has a stipend or because a close friend is applying there as well. Keep your long-term goals in mind and strategize on how you can best achieve them.

Step 4: Become Familiar with The Dietetic Internship Centralized Application System (DICAS)

Most dietetic internships now use the Dietetic Internship Centralized Application System or DICAS for handling internship applications. Applications are submitted through DICAS between specific dates and times for each internship appointment period. See http://www.eatright.org/ACEND /content.aspx?id=6442453138 for further information on DICAS.[9] Coordinated programs do not participate in DICAS or in computer matching.

Step 5: Register for Computer Matching

Computer matching is the process by which internship placement decisions are made. The computer matching for dietetic internships is handled by D & D Digital (http://www.dnddigital.com/).[10] While CPs and Dietetic Technician programs have their own applicant-selection processes, students who are applying for post-baccalaureate DIs participate in national computer matching for internship placement. A few internships do not participate in computer matching because they accept only graduates of their sponsoring institution. (For example, a university-sponsored internship accepts applications only from graduates of that university's DPD program.) Otherwise, all other internships must participate in the computer-matching process.

Computer matching is a contractual agreement between the Academy and D & D Digital Systems, whereby you are matched through a computerized process with the highest-ranked program that offers you a position. Computer matching uses the prioritized list of programs to which you applied and the internship's prioritized list of their applicants to make the matches. There is a $50 charge to applicants to participate in this process.

Much thought should be given to prioritizing the programs to which you have applied. You must remember that your highest priority match is the one you must accept, so this step is a very important one. You register and prioritize your internship choices online at the D & D Digital website. Once you have prioritized your applications, be sure to keep a copy for your records.

Step 6: Seek Letters of Reference/Recommendations

Pay attention to the program's requirements for letters of reference or recommendations. Also be aware of the Family Educational Rights and Privacy Act (FERPA), which requires that you give permission for a faculty member to release information about you, such as your grade point average, class rank, and other specific information that is not part of your public records.[11] Check with your university about how they are ensuring that FERPA requirements are being followed.

Be professional in your approach when asking individuals to write references or recommendations for you. Do not wait until the last minute! Many didactic program directors and other faculty members are inundated with requests for letters and recommendations by students who are all applying to supervised practice programs at the same time. It is critical that you provide as much information as possible to this person so that he or she can write an accurate and insightful recommendation for you. One idea might be to provide the recommendation writer a copy of your application to the program. At minimum, you should provide a current résumé. Give a specific date by which you need to have the recommendations completed, allowing a little extra time so that if the individual falls behind in the task, you won't be late in meeting the application deadline.

As part of your DICAS application procedure, you will be asked to provide the names and email addresses of individuals providing references for you. These individuals will be sent an email with instructions on how to submit their recommendations for you online through the DICAS process.

Step 7: Send Official Transcripts of All Academic Coursework

Official transcripts of your academic coursework from all colleges and universities you have attended must be submitted as part of the DICAS process. "Official" transcripts are in sealed envelopes, are stamped with the seal of the university, and are typically mailed directly from the university registrar's office to the address you designate. If you attended multiple schools, remember that you must obtain transcripts from all schools, and you must allow time for this process. Official copies of transcripts are mailed to the DICAS Transcript Department, P.O. Box 9118, Watertown, MA 02472, to become part of your centralized application.

Step 8: Proofread Your Application

Have your dietetics program director and/or academic advisor proofread a draft of your application. Remember that your application is likely the only representation the internship will have of you. Grammatical mistakes and typographical errors may make the difference in whether your application is rated lower than someone else's. The smallest things can make a huge difference in your success.

Step 9: Make a Copy of Your Application

Make a copy of your application for your files. It is always important for you to keep a copy of such important documents in case of computer system malfunction or some other unforeseen circumstance.

Step 10: Check the Due Date

Check the date when the applications are due. Typically, this date is in mid-February for a fall supervised practice start date or mid-September for a January start date. If you are applying to a graduate program as well as to the supervised practice program, check the deadlines for this application, because the dates may be different.

The Interview as Part of the Admission Process

Some supervised practice programs may include an interview as part of the admission process. Often this is a telephone interview. Prepare for this interview as you would for a job interview. Check the date and time for the interview and be punctual. Before the interview, make a list of questions you would like to ask, and think through questions that might be posed to you. Take the call in a quiet location where you will not be interrupted. Also, consider taking the call on a "corded phone" rather than on a cell phone, where you might lose the signal or otherwise get disconnected. Remember to smile while you are talking. It shows in your voice! Be enthusiastic and upbeat. Even though the interview committee can't see you, they will be able to sense the energy and excitement in your voice.

Match Day for Dietetic Internship Placement

The day on which you find out if you have matched for an internship placement is one filled with anticipation and excitement. The dates for "Match Day" are announced by the Academy and D & D Digital Systems each year. Your DPD director can provide this information for you. Students who apply for a DI starting in the fall are notified of the match results on a specific "Notification Day" in April. Students applying for a DI starting in the spring are notified on a "Notification Day" in November.

Before the notification date arrives, you will be sent specific login information and a password so that you can access the D & D Digital website at the specified date and time to see the results of the computer-matching process.

What happens if you do not receive a match? It's not the end of the world. Sometimes programs do not fill all their available internship slots. D & D Digital will post on its website a list of programs that have open internships and want those openings advertised. If you give permission, your name and contact information will be sent to these internships and to your DPD director. Your DPD director can work with you to look at the internships that have open positions and evaluate whether you'd like to submit your application to one of those programs. Each year, many students who did not receive a match in the computer process eventually receive an internship placement in this "secondary" process. Or, you may elect to wait until the next round of computer matching and reapply.

Once you have finished your academic program, your DPD director will provide you with a Verification Statement indicating that you have completed your final DPD coursework. Your DPD director must sign this form, and you must send it to your internship director before starting the supervised practice experience. Pack your bags! You're on your way!

Being Successful in the Supervised Practice Experience

Whether you are participating in a DI, a CP, or a Dietetic Technician program, the supervised practice experience is one of the most exciting times in your professional preparation. It is vital that you take advantage of every learning opportunity during this critical time. The following are some things to keep in mind during your supervised practice experience:

- Establish a cordial and cooperative relationship with your preceptor(s) and share your interests and professional goals. Look at this internship experience as if you were beginning a new job. Always look and act professionally as a member of the organization's team. Remember that you are still learning. Confidence is a good thing, but do not act like you know all the answers!

- Come to your experience prepared to take advantage of this wonderful opportunity you've been given. Do your "homework" before each learning experience by reviewing your notes and looking over readings that relate to that rotation. Before you begin each day, formulate objectives and think through what you want to accomplish. At the end of the day, do a quick assessment of how successful you were in reaching your goals, and reformulate new goals for the following day.

- Remember "the big picture" and use systems thinking. Do not get so engrossed in one activity that you miss what else is going on around you. Analyze what you are doing and how it relates to everything else in your unit, department, or to the organization as a whole. Every decision or action has repercussions throughout the organization. Take time to make those connections and learn from them.

- Plan your time wisely and accomplish as much as you can. If you are in the middle of an important task with which you have been charged, finish the task. Others may be depending on your completion of that assignment. Remember that professionals often are salaried, not hourly, employees. Stay until the job is done and your responsibilities have been fulfilled. Do not be a "clock watcher"!

- Be flexible, positive, enthusiastic, and polite. Demonstrate initiative, but remember there are limits to your authority. If you're not sure what those boundaries are, check with your preceptor. And finally, treat others the way you'd want to be treated. Remember that the professionals you work within your supervised practice experience may be references for you for future employment or other opportunities. Do not burn any bridges!

When Supervised Practice Is Completed

Completion of your supervised practice experience signifies the end of the second step in the three-step process of becoming a credentialed dietetics professional. If you are a CP or Dietetic Technician Program student, one Verification Statement will be issued to you, showing that you have completed both the academic and supervised practice requirements to sit for the national credentialing exam. CP students are eligible to take the national Registration Examination for Dietitians, whereas Dietetic Technician graduates are eligible for the national Registration Examination for Dietetic Technicians.

For individuals completing a DI, a second Verification Statement will be provided showing that the intern has met the supervised practice requirements. This statement will be added to the academic Verification Statement from the DPD program, thus indicating that all requirements are met and that the individual is ready to move to step 3, sitting for the national Registration Examination for Dietitians.

Supervised practice provides the required hands-on work experience for you to be ready for the national credentialing examination as a dietetics professional. It is a time of hard work and learning, networking and growth, excitement and promise. The people you meet and work with during this time are vital mentors for your professional growth. Take advantage of gaining everything you can from the experience, and when you are a dietetics professional perhaps you'll have the opportunity to guide the supervised practice experience for another aspiring professional!

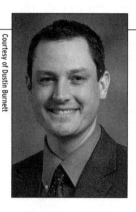

Courtesy of Dustin Burnett

Profile of a Professional

Dustin J. Burnett, MS, RD

Principal Dietitian, Supervisor
Metabolic Kitchen and Human Feeding Lab
Western Human Nutrition Research Center
United States Department of Agriculture
University of California–Davis, California

Education:
Culinary Certification, Grossmont College, El Cajon, California
AS in Chemistry, City College of San Francisco, California
BS in Nutrition/Dietetics and Toxicology–University of California, Berkeley
Dietetic Internships, Tufts Medical Center/Frances Stern Nutrition Center, Boston, Massachusetts
MS in Clinical Nutrition, Tufts University/Friedman School of Nutrition Science and Policy, Boston, Massachusetts

How did you first hear about dietetics and decide to become a Registered Dietitian?
I took a basic nutrition course as a requirement for the culinary arts program in which I was enrolled full time at a community college. The dietitian who taught the course drew the structure of beta-carotene on the board, and I was enamored. When she explained what a free radical was, I was convinced that I needed to be studying chemistry. I took my culinary certificates and transferred into the chemistry department, where I earned my associate of science degree in chemistry. From there, I began the path to earn my bachelor of science in toxicology. It was at this level where I took physiology and made friends with some of the dietetics majors. I learned about the diversity of their coursework; that is, pure sciences, economics, psychology, accounting, culture, counseling, food science, pathophysiology, organizational behavior, and so on. I soon made the decision that studying dietetics would help me develop a more diversified skill set than lab work; it would provide me with the skills that are needed in the modern business world. The rest, as they say, is history!

What kind of work experiences did you have while you were in school?
While pursuing my education, I became involved with student government and took on a number of volunteering opportunities. I was also employed the entire time I was in college. I worked as a meat and seafood clerk in a supermarket (e.g., developed supermarket savvy, learned the various cuts of meats and poultry, developed people skills), a barista in an urban coffeehouse (e.g., developed "street smarts," learned how to manage people, and had all the coffee I wanted), a diet clerk in a residential senior complex (e.g., learned tray line, forecasting techniques, tallying, a variety of therapeutic diets, and learned how to communicate with the elder community), and a diet

assistant in a general clinical research center—this is where I found home! This is where I fit in because I naturally focus on the process more than the results. My philosophy is this: if the process is clearly defined, then good results will surely follow. Of course, no system is perfect.

What are some examples of your professional involvement?

Bay Area Dietetic Association (BADA)—Student Liaison and Representative
Massachusetts Student Dietetic Association (MSDA)—Vice President
Member of the Academy of Nutrition and Dietetics, the Food and Culinary Professional Practice Group and the Research Practice Group

What excites you about dietetics and the future of our profession?

Our field is continually changing, and it's difficult to "paint yourself into a corner." If you are the type of person who thrives in a world of learning and skill development, you will not be bored. The dietetics profession prepares you for the real world. You will develop skills in a variety of areas. You may not make as much money as, say, a banker or financier, but if you put forth honest, genuine collaborative effort, you will have a job that is very rewarding and you will look forward to showing up to work.

Why/how is teamwork important to you in your position? How have you been involved in team projects?

Teamwork drives my very existence as a dietitian. No one person has all of the information needed to perform a job correctly. At work, I am a member of the Health and Safety Team, which oversees the safety of the employees, interns, and study participants. I'm also a member of the Human Studies Committee, which oversees all of the current and future human studies that will occur at the Center. I collaborate with the university professors to establish teaching criteria for internship rotations. I collaborate with other centers to develop food safety guidelines and nutrition resources for the general public. I assist with the USDA booth at the Academy of Nutrition and Dietetic's annual Food and Nutrition Conference and Expo, and the list goes on. If one is not able to serve as a member of a team, then one will have a difficult time making it in the professional world of dietetics. It is a fundamental skill. Learn to get excited about group work!

What words of wisdom do you have for future dietetics professionals?

Find your passion, because it will carry you through tough times. Also remember that passion is a double-edged sword; do not let it cloud your rational thinking. Always remind yourself that there is both the "ideal world" and the "real world" and they are rarely ever the same.

- No matter whatever responsibilities you take on, do your absolute best.
- Do not give up, and if you feel like you are struggling, it's probably because you are really learning.
- Do not compare yourself to others, and do not try to be someone else (you will always be an imitation)!
- Start with what interests you, and then find what it is that makes your brain "tick."
- Know what you are good at, and also what you are not good at.
- Do not get discouraged if someone tells you something you do not want to hear.
- Do not always do what comes natural to you; if you do, you are not learning or expanding your knowledge. Remember, you've got to dig the trenches, lay the foundation, and build the structure before you get to decorate and enjoy your new home.

Remember, "Nutrition is a science; not a religion. It is based upon matters of fact; not questions of belief."

—Stephen Barrett, MD, and Victor Herbert, MD, JD

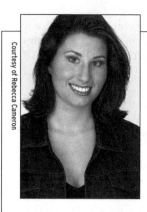

Profile of a Professional

Rebecca Cameron, RD

Chef, Chandy's Natural Café
Sole Proprietor, Haute Nutrition
Redmond, Washington

Education:
BS in Food and Nutrition, Seattle Pacific University, Seattle,
    Washington
Dietetic Internship, Sea Mar Community Health Center,
    Seattle, Washington
AS in Culinary Arts, Culinary Institute of America, Hyde Park,
    New York

How did you first learn about dietetics as a profession?
I grew up in a household that was very nutrition conscious. My mom cooked very healthy meals and encouraged us to try new foods. Once I entered high school, I took a health class and was fascinated by the way vitamins/minerals work in the human body. When I discovered I could have a career as a Registered Dietitian, I chose my college based on the nutrition program that was offered.

What was your route to registration as a dietitian?
I applied to internships during my senior year of college. I had been researching the programs for several years, so I was pretty sure that I had narrowed the choices down to a good match. I also attended a few open houses around the country to assist me in my decision-making process. I felt it was very helpful to personally meet with the program directors and see the actual internship site. I was fortunate to be selected by Sea Mar Community Health Center in Seattle for my internship experience.

Describe your career path thus far.
I started my career in clinical nutrition at one of the hospitals I rotated through during my internship. I felt it was important to have a good foundation in clinical nutrition before branching out into other areas of nutrition. I always knew that I would end up in a culinary-related position. After a year, I accepted a position as part of the food team for a corporate food manufacturer. My work consisted of supporting our chef with nutrition analysis and quality assurance initiatives. After working in this field for several years, I left to attend culinary school to receive a formal culinary education.

My culinary education gave me the education and training necessary to formulate a business that concentrates on bridging culinary arts with nutrition. I began by providing the service of ingredient statements and nutrition analyses to restaurants and food manufacturers. Gradually, this grew into research and development to meet guidelines for nutrition content claims on labels. Eventually, I decided to become the chef for a restaurant that I helped conceptualize. At Chandy's Natural Café, I provide a range of nutrition-focused menu items using local ingredients whenever possible.

What are some examples of your professional involvement?
Throughout my career I have been active in my local dietetic association as a student recruiter, then later as a media coordinator. Over the years, I have volunteered with a variety of food and culinary associations in positions ranging from assisting with annual meetings to newsletter editing.

Have you received honors or awards?
I received the Management Award upon graduation from the Culinary Institute of America. In 2007, I was honored to be selected to serve on the CIA Alumni Council.

How is teamwork important to you in your position?

Teamwork is a daily part of working in a kitchen and collaborating with a variety of professionals in the restaurant business. In order for a restaurant operation to be successful, there has to be teamwork. It's essentially the glue of the business. My work requires teamwork with disciplines such as marketing, operations, purchasing, and management.

What words of wisdom do you have for future dietetics professionals?

I'm excited that the role of nutrition is emerging as a focus in so many career areas. For example, in culinary arts, recognition of the role of nutrition is growing rapidly due to such factors as the obesity epidemic, the move to reduce trans fats, and the emphasis on sustainable foods. In clinical nutrition, the dietitian's role is moving toward a variety of specializations. Dietitians are even placing feeding tubes and assisting with diagnosis of food insensitivities. The range of career opportunities within the field of dietetics has always excited me, and now that range is growing ever broader.

Take advantage of the opportunities given to you, such as volunteering, job shadowing, assisting a professor, or other types of work experience. Take advantage of every opportunity now while you have the time to do so. The contacts made now are very likely to benefit you in the future.

Suggested Activities

1. Interview someone who is currently involved in a supervised practice experience or who has completed one recently. Ask the person about his or her experiences, including likes and dislikes about the supervised practice experience. Ask for his or her advice as you consider the application process.

2. Look at the list of core competencies for supervised practice for DTRs or RDs on the Academy website. How do these competencies relate to the "Core Knowledge" acquired during the didactic process?

3. Study the verbs used in the core competency statements. What do these indicate about the job activities of entry-level dietetics professionals?

4. Talk to someone who has just finished the supervised practice experience. Ask the individual to describe one of the best learning experiences and explain why the experience was so meaningful. What was a difficult learning experience, and what did the person bring away from that experience?

5. Complete a self-assessment plan.

   a. Go to the Academy website or look at a copy of the *Applicant Guide to Supervised Practice Experiences*, and identify three supervised practice programs in which you might be interested.

   b. Find out as much as you can about the supervised practice program through its webpage, printed material, or by contacting the program director for more information. Complete a written summary of each of the supervised practice programs. Make sure to include the following information:

    i. Number of students/interns applying

    ii. Number of applicants accepted in the last 2 years

    iii. Minimum GPA required

    iv. Average GPA of current students

    v. Length of the supervised practice program

    vi. Full-time program or part-time options?

    vii. What rotations are included in the program, where are the training sites, and how long are the rotations?

    viii. What is the cost of attending the program?

    ix. GRE required for admission?

    x. Option to obtain an advanced degree along with the supervised practice experience?

    xi. Other requirements for program admission, such as work experience or volunteer experience?

    xii. Interview required? If so, is it an in-person interview or a phone interview?

c. Summarize what these programs are looking for and how applicants are evaluated. Identify at least three criteria that are considered.

d. On each of these criteria, assess your own readiness on a scale of 1 to 10, with 1 being "needs a lot of work" and 10 being "outstanding."

e. Describe your readiness for the supervised practice experience, and justify the scores you gave yourself on the different criteria.

f. Design a plan and describe, in detail, what you can do to increase or maintain your scores so you can maximize your chances of being accepted into a supervised practice program.

Selected Websites

- www.eatright.org/BecomeanRDorDTR/content.aspx?id=8156—Academy of Nutrition and Dietetics list of all accredited supervised practice programs
- www.eatright.org/BecomeanRDorDTR/content.aspx?id=8473—Academy of Nutrition and Dietetics lists the DIs that operate by distance education
- www.eatright.org/BecomeanRDorDTR/default.aspx—Academy of Nutrition and Dietetics Student Center
- www.eatright.org/uploadedFiles/CADE/CADE-General-Content/3-08_DT-FKC_Only.pdf—Competency statements for Dietetic Technician programs
- www.eatright.org/uploadedFiles/CADE/CADE-General-Content/3-08_RD-FKC_Only.pdf—Competency statements for RD programs

- www.dnddigital.com—D & D Digital
- www.depdpg.org—DI application form
- www.depdpg.org—Nutrition and Dietetics Educators and Preceptors Dietetic Practice Group

References

1. Academy of Nutrition and Dietetics. 2012 ACEND Standards for Dietitian Education Programs. Available at http://www.eatright.org/ACEND/content.aspx?id=7877. Accessed May 18, 2012.

2. Academy of Nutrition and Dietetics. ACEND 2012 Standards for Technician Education Programs. http://www.eatright.org/ACEND/content.aspx?id=7877. Accessed May 18, 2012.

3. Academy of Nutrition and Dietetics. Coordinated Programs in Dietetics. Available at: http://www.eatright.org/ACEND/content.aspx?id=74. Accessed May 18, 2012.

4. Nutrition and Dietetic Educators and Preceptors. Available at: http://www.depdpg.org/. Accessed May 5, 2012.

5. Academy of Nutrition and Dietetics. Internships. Available at: http://www.eatright.org/BecomeanRDorDTR/content.aspx?id=8147. Accessed May 5, 2012.

6. Academy of Nutrition and Dietetics. Dietetic Internships: Programs Offering Distance Education. Available at: http://www.eatright.org/BecomeanRDorDTR/content.aspx?id=8473. Accessed May 5, 2012.

7. Individualized Supervised Practice Pathways (ISPPs). http://www.eatright.org/ACEND/content.aspx?id=6442465002. Accessed May 18, 2012.

8. Academy of Nutrition and Dietetics. Accredited Education Programs. Available at: http://www.eatright.org/BecomeanRDorDTR/content.aspx?id=8156. Accessed May 5, 2012.

9. Nutrition and Dietetic Educators and Preceptors. Dietetic Internship Program Application. Available at: http://www.depdpg.org. Accessed May 5, 2012.

10. D & D Digital. Academy of Nutrition and Dietetics Internship Matching. http://www.dnddigital.com/. Accessed May 18, 2012.

11. U.S. Department of Education. Family Educational Rights and Privacy Act (FERPA). Available at: http://www2.ed.gov/policy/gen/guid/fpco/ferpa/index.html. Accessed January 25, 2010.

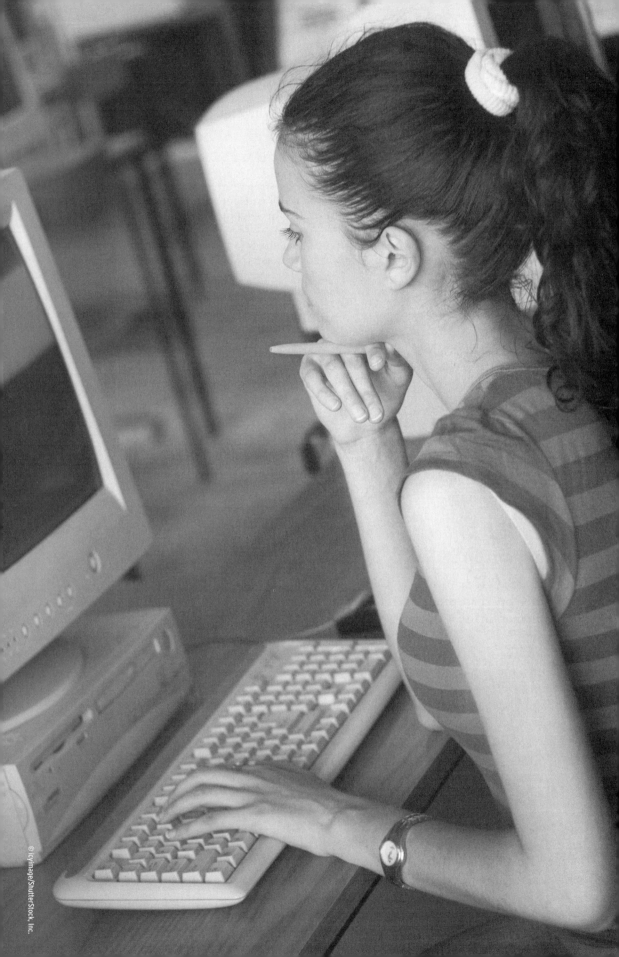

Credentialing

Protecting the Public

Defining the competence required of practitioners is an important quality-assurance activity for any profession. According to *Webster's Dictionary*, the word *credential* means "a letter or certificate given to a person to show that he has a right to confidence or to the exercise of a certain position or authority; that which gives credit; that which entitles to credit, confidence, etc., establishing reliability."[1] This is an appropriate description of the work of the Commission on Dietetic Registration (CDR).

Commission on Dietetic Registration

The CDR, the credentialing arm of the Academy, was first called the Committee on Professional Registration. In 1969, it was charged with the implementation of national dietetic registration. In November 1975, the CDR was made an independent unit of the ADA. The CDR is responsible for all aspects of the registration process: standard setting for registration eligibility, examination development and administration, credentialing, and recertification. The CDR grants recognition of entry-level competence to dietitians who meet its standards and qualifications. These dietitians may use the legally protected professional designation *Registered Dietitian*, or the initials RD. Dietetic technicians who meet the standards and qualifications for technicians may use the legally protected professional designation *Dietetic Technician, Registered*, or the initials DTR.

The Commission consists of 11 members. Credentialed practitioners, RDs and DTRs, elect nine members. These include seven RDs, one RD specialist, and one DTR. A newly credentialed practitioner is appointed by the Commission for a 1-year term. In addition, a public representative is appointed to the Commission and has full rights and privileges.[2]

Dietetic Registration

The purpose of registration is to protect the nutritional health, safety, and welfare of the public by encouraging high standards of performance of individuals practicing in the profession of dietetics.[3] Registration of dietitians began in 1969, providing a legally protected title for credentialed practitioners. At its inception, registration required membership in the ADA, completion of an examination, and a continuing education requirement. More than 19,000 members of the ADA were "grandfathered" and became registered during the initial enrollment period when the examination was waived.[3] As of 2011, there were 81,619 RDs.[4] Dietetic technicians were first admitted to membership in the ADA in 1975. Certification for DTRs became a reality in 1983. The CDR currently recognizes 4,237 DTRs.[4] Membership in the Academy is not a requirement for RD or DTR status.

The Registration Examination

The development of the examinations for RD and DTR status is rigorous. **Figure 7–1** outlines the steps in the CDR's test development program.

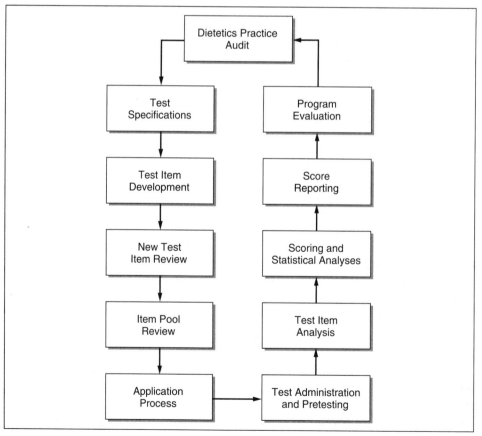

FIGURE 7–1 Certification testing program.
Courtesy of Commission on Dietetic Registration, Academy of Nutrition and Dietetics, Chicago, IL

The **dietetics practice audit** is the important first step in this process. A practice audit is an in-depth study of dietetics practice that describes the knowledge and skills needed to perform in a competent manner at a specified level of dietetics practice.

From the practice audit, a blueprint for building the examination must be developed. **Test specifications** include a description of the content to be tested, the proportion of the test to be devoted to various content areas, and the characteristics of acceptable test items. Because the test specifications come from the dietetics practice audit, the test is deemed to be valid and credible.

Test item development is an exciting but time-consuming experience. Individuals trained in the specifics of test construction develop test questions. Care is taken in choosing individuals who represent diverse practice areas and population subgroups. Four criteria are applied to each test question: (1) the question must be relevant and critical to entry-level practice; (2) the question must be accurate, current, and clear; (3) the question must not reflect regional or institutional differences; and (4) the question must conform to test specifications. Test items are reviewed by professional test editors to eliminate technical flaws, ambiguities, and potential bias. Questions that are considered to be editorially and technically sound are then pretested as unscored items on an actual exam. Such a "trial run" of the unscored items allows the test developers to see whether the test item truly discriminates between those who are entry-level competent and those who are not.

During the **item pool review** process, experienced test reviewers appointed by the CDR review the items for content accuracy, currency, and relevance to entry-level practice. They must also be sure that each item has one best answer. Only when a test item has successfully passed the content, measurement, and editorial review, will that item be included in the computer-based test item pool.

After each test item has been pretested as an unscored item, psychometricians perform **test item analysis**. Performance statistics are reviewed for each test question to identify problems. Experienced item writers review test items that appear to be problematic before those items are included in the scored item pool. This eliminates items with potential response problems or ambiguities. This review process is repeated on an ongoing basis as test items are administered.

The CDR periodically conducts a **passing-score determination study**, using experienced dietetics professionals from diverse practice areas and population subgroups. Content experts establish the minimum level of acceptable professional performance expected on a certification test. The CDR uses a criterion-referenced approach for determining the passing score. This criterion-referenced passing score becomes the basis for equating future exams, thus ensuring that all the versions of the examinations are of equal level of difficulty.

Score reporting announces the examinee's performance on the certification exam. The report gives a total scaled score as well as sub-scaled scores in the different test domains (nutrition and foodservice). Twice a year, in February and August, the CDR provides dietetic education programs with both a test summary of how the institution's graduates have performed and also individual scores by name when the examinee has authorized his or her scores to be released to the program.[5]

Computer-Adaptive Testing

Since July 1999 computers have administered registration examinations for both RDs and DTRs. The CDR decided to implement computerized testing because it recognized the many advantages this method offers to examinees. These include the following:

- Flexible test administration dates allow examinees to schedule the examination at a time convenient to them throughout the year.
- Retesting is available 45 days after the previous test date.
- A unique examination is generated based on each examinee's entry-level competence.
- Score reports are distributed to examinees as they leave the test site.

The registration examinations are administered at specified ACT test sites nationwide. Eligible candidates can call the nearest participating ACT test site to schedule an appointment to take the examination. The cost for the *Registration Examination for Dietitians* is $200 and $120 for the *Registration Examination for Dietetic Technicians*.

The examinations are variable in length. For the RD examination, each test taker is given a *minimum* of 125 questions; 100 of these are scored questions and 25 are questions that are being pretested for use on subsequent examinations and are unscored. The *maximum* number of questions possible is 145; 120 are scored questions and 25 are unscored pretest questions.

For the DTR examination, each examinee is given a *minimum* of 110 questions; 80 of these are scored questions and 30 are unscored pretest questions. The *maximum* number of questions is 130, with 100 scored items and 30 unscored pretest items. All questions for either the RD or DTR exam are in multiple-choice format.

For both examinations, test takers are given a total of 3 hours, which includes time for an introductory tutorial. The clock starts ticking with the administration of the first test question. From that point, the test taker has a maximum of 2.5 hours to finish the exam. The test taker has the option of having the "time remaining" show on the screen. If watching those numbers click down is a distraction, you can hide the clock!

If you've never taken a computer-based examination, you should practice taking such a test. Note that on the computerized examination once a question is presented you must answer that question. You cannot skip to the next question or go back and change an answer. You must answer each question as it comes and then move to the next one.

The CDR has prepared two study guides, one for the RD exam and one for the DTR exam. Both guides provide a comprehensive study outline, references, and a practice examination. A practice exam is available in both the printed and online versions of the study guide. The practice examination in the online version simulates the actual computerized registration examination format. You may purchase the study guides from the Academy by calling 1-800-877-1600, ext. 5000. Alternatively, you may purchase the study guides by visiting the Academy Marketplace online (see www.eatright .org). The cost of either study guide is $65.

Individuals who have completed both the academic preparation and the supervised practice requirements and have received signed Verification Statements for both of these experiences may sit for the national *Registration Examination for Dietitians* or the *Registration Examination for Dietetic Technicians*. A Verification Statement signed by the program director and a transcript documenting completion of the required courses must be submitted with the examination application. If a person is returning to college or university to complete a degree started at some earlier time, a dietetics program may require that person to update previous coursework before issuing a Verification Statement. You should check with the dietetics program director to find out about such program requirements. Once your eligibility to take the examination has been established, you will be sent a letter that authorizes you to schedule an examination time with ACT. This authorization document expires 1 year after its issuance. If you don't successfully complete the RD or DTR exam within 1 year, you must contact CDR to be reauthorized.[5]

Getting Ready for the Credentialing Examination

The credentialing exam is the culmination of all your years of hard work and study. Preparing to take the exam can be a stressful time, and the examination may come at a very busy time. Perhaps you've just graduated or finished your supervised practice experience. Perhaps you're starting a new job, or you've just moved or gotten married or any other of the many life-changing experiences that may be happening as you move into your career. Finding time to organize and review your material may be a challenge, but it is a critical activity! No one should ever walk into the credentialing examination without lots of study and preparation.

As mentioned in the previous section, the CDR produces study guides for both the RD and DTR examinations, and these publications are an excellent place to start the review process. However, you may wish to pursue other study activities. Several entrepreneurs have established workshops that help individuals organize and review for the RD exam. Some of these also have printed study materials that are included in the registration fee to attend the workshop. Some sell these materials separately for study on your own. These RD exam review sessions may last 2–3 days and are held in various parts of the country. Check with your program director or look in the back of the *Journal of the Academy of Nutrition and Dietetics* for further information. Examples include the reviews by Breeding & Associates[6] or Inman Seminars.[7] Program directors are often sent brochures about these review sessions and can share this information with you. Some dietetic education programs also provide review sessions for their own graduates and your program director will let you know if this service is available.

Other entrepreneurs have developed other media to help examinees study for the credentialing exam. Two examples are "RD in a Flash" flash cards[8] and DietitianExam.com, an online study program.[9] Before you pay for any kind of review material or program, ask the following questions to help you make a more informed decision:

- How long have you been in business?
- How many people have used your service?
- What is the pass rate on the RD exam of those people who have used your service?
- Would you share with me some names and contact information of individuals who have used your service?
- When did you last update your review materials?
- Do you have simulated computer-based testing as part of your service?

Taking the credentialing examination is a stressful experience. Before the scheduled time for your examination, keep the following in mind:

- Get a good night's sleep the night before the exam.
- Confirm the time and location of the exam.
- Allow yourself plenty of time to get to the testing site. If you do not arrive on time, the test will have to be rescheduled.
- Make sure you arrive with a photo ID for identification purposes.
- A calculator will be provided for you at the test site. Don't try taking your own; you won't be allowed to use it.
- If you encounter a computer malfunction during the exam, you will be asked to wait 45 minutes while the problem is investigated. If it is not possible to resolve the problem in this time frame, you will be rescheduled to retest as soon as possible.
- Remember, if you don't pass the exam, it's not the end of the world! You may retake the exam as soon as 45 days later. Review your materials and try again.
- When you pass, celebrate by sharing the good news with your didactic program director and your supervised practice program director.

Maintaining Registered Status

Continuing education has always been an integral part of professional registration. As the profession of dietetics continues to change and expand into new areas of practice, it is vital that dietetics professionals be lifelong learners. As we move into new and uncharted waters, each of us must update and broaden our knowledge base for effective dietetics practice. The CDR was one of the first health-related credentialing agencies to insist on continuing education. To maintain registered status, dietetics professionals must document their participation in professional development activities by creating a Professional Development Portfolio (PDP). During each 5-year reporting period, RDs must achieve 75 continuing professional education units (CPEUs), and DTRs must achieve 50 CPEUs. The CPEUs must be based on each person's individual learning needs as identified in the professional development portfolio process.

Steps in Professional Portfolio Development

The steps in developing one's portfolio are as follows:

- Reflect on your professional practice to establish professional goals.
- Conduct a learning needs assessment to identify what you know now and what you need to learn to reach your goals.
- Develop a learning plan that shows how you will meet your goals.
- Implement your learning plan through continuing professional development activities.
- Evaluate your learning plan outcomes to assess how you have applied what you've learned and its impact on reaching your goals, refocusing those goals when necessary.

The CDR defines *continuing education* as education beyond that required for entry into the profession. Educational programs may apply directly to the field of nutrition and dietetics or they may launch the learner into new areas such as computer technology, physical assessment, or marketing. Whatever the learning activity, it should update or enhance one's knowledge and skills for new applications in dietetics practice. Some examples of continuing education activities include:

- Lectures
- Workshops
- Journal clubs and study groups
- Seminars
- Case presentations
- Video, audio, and computer-based materials
- Self-study programs
- Culinary skills training
- Physical assessment training
- Multi-skill training
- Computer technology training[10]

Specialty Credentials

In 1993, the first specialty examinations were administered, enabling RDs who met the prescribed criteria to become board certified in specific specialty areas of dietetics practice. Currently, the CDR offers specialty credentials in five areas:

- Board Certified Specialist in Renal Nutrition (CSR)
- Board Certified Specialist in Pediatric Nutrition (CSP)
- Board Certified Specialist in Sports Dietetics (CSSD)
- Board Certified Specialist in Gerontological Nutrition (CSG)
- Board Certified Specialist in Oncology Nutrition (CSO)

These credentials typically require that the candidate have been an RD for at least 2 years and have from 1,500 to 2,000 hours of practice in the area of specialty. The schedules of when and where examinations will be administered are announced each year by the CDR. Criteria for eligibility to sit for the examinations and other details about each credential may be found online at www.cdrnet.org/certifications.[11] As of 2011, there were 412 CSRs, 519 CSPs, 415 CSSDs, 319 CSGs, and 370 CSOs.[12]

Specialty credentials are also available from other professional organizations. Some of these certifications are listed in **Table 7–1**.

TABLE 7–1

Health- and Fitness-Related Credentials

Credential	Contact Information
ACE Certified Clinical Exercise Specialist	American Council on Exercise 4851 Paramount Drive, San Diego, CA 92123 Phone: 800-825-3636 Email: *support@acefitness.org*
ACE Certified Group Fitness Instructor	American Council on Exercise 4851 Paramount Drive, San Diego, CA 92123 Phone: 800-825-3636 Email: *support@acefitness.org*
ACE Certified Lifestyle & Weight Management Consultant	American Council on Exercise 4851 Paramount Drive, San Diego, CA 92123 Phone: 800-825-3636 Email: *support@acefitness.org*
ACE Certified Personal Trainer	American Council on Exercise 4851 Paramount Drive, San Diego, CA 92123 Phone: 800-825-3636 Email: *support@acefitness.org*
ACSM Certified Exercise Specialist Instructor	American College of Sports Medicine P.O. Box 1440 Indianapolis, IN 46206-1440 Phone: 317-637-9200 Email: *certification@acsm.org*
ACSM Certified Health/Fitness Instructor	American College of Sports Medicine P.O. Box 1440 Indianapolis, IN 46206-1440 Phone: 317-637-9200 Email: *certification@acsm.org*
ACSM Registered Clinical Exercise Physiologist	American College of Sports Medicine P.O. Box 1440 Indianapolis, IN 46206-1440 Phone: 317-637-9200 Email: *certification@acsm.org*
Board Certified in Advanced Diabetes Management	American Association of Diabetes Educators 200 W. Madison Street, Suite 800 Chicago, IL 60606 Phone: 800-338-3633
Certified Clinical Nutritionist (CCN)	International and American Associations of Clinical Nutritionists (IAACN) 15280 Addison Road, Suite 130 Addison, TX 75001 Phone: 972-407-9089

Certified Diabetes Educator (CDE)	National Certification Board for Diabetes Educators 330 E. Algonquin Road, Suite 4 Arlington Heights, IL 60005 Phone: 847-228-9795
Certified in Family and Consumer Sciences (CFCS)	American Association of Family and Consumer Sciences 400 N. Columbus Street, Suite 202 Alexandria, VA 22314 Phone: 703-706-4600
Certified Foodservice Professional (CFSP)	North American Association of Food Equipment Manufacturers 161 N. Clark Street, Suite 2020 Chicago, IL 60601 Phone: 312-821-0201
Certified Health Education Specialist (CHES)	National Commission for Health Education Credentialing, Inc. 1541 Alta Drive, Suite 303 Whitehall, PA 18052-5642 Phone: 800-813-0727
Certified Nutrition Specialist (CNS)	Certification Board of Nutrition Specialists of the American College of Nutrition 300 S. Duncan Avenue, Suite 225 Clearwater, FL 33755 Phone: 727-446-6086
Certified Nutrition Support Clinician (CNSC)	National Board of Nutrition Support Certification, Inc., of the American Society for Parenteral and Enteral Nutrition 8630 Fenton Street, Suite 412 Silver Spring, MD 20910 Phone: 301-587-6315 or 800-727-4567
Certified Professional in Healthcare Quality	Healthcare Quality Certification Board of the National Association for Healthcare Quality 18000 W. 105th Street Olathe, KS 66061-7543 Phone: 913-895-4609
International Board Certified Lactation Consultant, Registered Lactation Consultant (IBCLC, RLC)	International Board of Lactation Consultant Examiners 6402 Arlington Boulevard, Suite 350 Falls Church, VA 22042 Phone: 703-560-7330
National Certified Counselor	National Board for Certified Counselors 3 Terrace Way, Suite D Greensboro, NC 27403-3660 Phone: 336-547-0607
School Foodservice and Nutrition Specialist (SFNS)	School Nutrition Association 700 S. Washington Street, Suite 300 Alexandria, VA 22314 Phone: 703-739-3900

Specialty credentials can be a valuable asset to the dietitian who holds them. Career advancement may be enhanced, salary levels may increase, and recognition of heightened expertise by other members of the healthcare team may be realized.

Fellow of the American Dietetic Association

The ADA established the credential *Fellow* to certify those registered dietitians who demonstrated empirically defined characteristics of achievement and leadership (abbreviated FADA, for Fellow of the ADA). To become a FADA, candidates must have met the following requirements:

- Be an RD.
- Submit documentation of a minimum of a master's degree, earned and granted by a regionally accredited U.S. college or university or foreign equivalent.
- Submit documentation of a minimum of 8 years' work experience as an RD.
- Submit documentation of at least one professional achievement.
- Submit documentation of professional positions.
- Submit documentation of professional contacts.
- Submit a written response to an approach-to-practice scenario.

A portfolio submitted by the candidate was judged through peer review. Certification as a FADA was granted for a 10-year period. During that period, fellows were required to maintain RD status and submit an annual maintenance fee. At this time, CDR is not accepting new applications for the FADA credential. However, you may meet RDs who have earned the FADA designation and continue to use this credential after their name.[13] Recommendation 8 in the "Final Report of the Phase 2 Future Dietetics Education and Practice Task Force" has recommended the reinstitution of an advanced-level practice credential in the future.[14]

Licensure

Licensure is "a state policy that provides consumers an assurance that a professional is competent to provide certain services and is used by professionals to exclude the nonlicensed from providing those services for a fee. It is a tool for creating and maintaining a verifiable minimum level of skill and competence."[15]

Licensure differs from registration in several ways. Although registration is recognized nationally, licensure is recognition by an individual state. Both credentialing systems afford some legal protection to the title of the practitioner, but licensure may also protect the right of an individual to practice in a state. Registration is voluntary, established and maintained in the private sector. Licensure may be either voluntary or mandatory, but it has formal legal status in the public sector.

At present, 46 states, the District of Columbia, and Puerto Rico have enacted some form of regulation. **Licensing statutes** include an explicitly defined scope of practice and make it illegal to practice dietetics without first obtaining a license from the state. **Statutory certification** limits the use of particular titles to persons meeting predetermined requirements, but persons not certified can still practice dietetics with a different title. **Registration** is the least restrictive form of state regulation. It prohibits use of the title *dietitian* by those not meeting state-mandated qualifications. However, unregistered persons may practice the profession.

Each state has a licensure contact person who can provide updates on professional regulation in that state. The name and telephone number of any state's licensure contact can be found on the CDR website (www.cdrnet.org).[16]

Other Tools Supporting Professional Competence

Evidence-Based Practice

According to the Academy, *evidence-based practice* is "the use of systematically reviewed scientific evidence in making food and nutrition practice decisions by integrating best available evidence with professional expertise and client values to improve outcomes."[17] The Academy has developed a plethora of resources to help dietetics professionals make practice decisions based on the best available scientific evidence. This evidence researches findings as well as national guidelines, policies, consensus statements, expert opinions, and quality improvement data.[17]

One of the most outstanding resources is the Academy's Evidence Analysis Library®. This resource, which is available free to Academy members, is a synthesis of the best, most relevant nutritional research on important dietetic practice questions in an accessible, online, user-friendly library.[18] The library covers a wide variety of topics including childhood overweight and obesity, nutritional counseling, critical illness, and so on. The database is consistently being updated and is available to members at any time.

Integrating research into daily dietetics practice is another important aspect of evidence-based practice. Dietetics professionals not only need to be informed of research going on in medical centers, universities, and so on, but also recognize that they can participate in research as part of their own dietetics practice. The Dietetics Practice-Based Research Network (DPBRN) brings together dietetics practitioners and researchers to identify and design research that can be carried out on the job.[19] Dietitians can propose ideas for research projects, serve on the advisory board that selects research projects to be pursued, help collect data on the job, and be a part of disseminating the research findings. You can find out more about the DPBRN on the Academy's website (www.eatright.org).

Standards of Practice and Standards of Professional Performance

The Standards of Practice (SOP) and Standards of Professional Performance (SOPPs) are tools for credentialed dietetics practitioners to use in professional development. They serve as guides for self-evaluation and to determine the education and skills needed to advance an individual's level of practice. Although not regulations, the standards may be used by regulatory agencies to determine competency for credentialed dietetics practitioners.[20]

The "American Dietetic Association Revised 2008 Standards of Practice in Nutrition Care and Standards of Professional Performance for Registered Dietitians and Dietetic Technicians, Registered" was published in the September 2008 issue of the *Journal of the American Dietetic Association*. These outline the minimum competent levels of practice for RDs and DTRs and serve as the core statements of professional competency. From this core, practice-specific SOPs and SOPPs have been developed. These practice-specific standards may be viewed on the Academy website (www.eatright.org).

The SOPs relate directly to patient care and are based on the four steps of the Nutrition Care Process (NCP):

- Nutrition Assessment
- Nutrition Diagnosis
- Nutrition Intervention
- Nutrition Monitoring and Evaluation

The SOPPs represent six domains of professionalism:

- Provision of Services
- Application of Research
- Communication and Application of Knowledge
- Utilization and Management of Resources
- Quality in Practice
- Competency and Accountability[20]

The SOPs and SOPPs are designed to be used for self-evaluation and can be used as part of the Professional Development Portfolio as each dietetic practitioner strives for ever-increasing levels of competence in his or her practice.

The Code of Ethics for the Profession of Dietetics

This enforceable code provides for public accountability by monitoring appropriate ethical performance by a dietetics practitioner and reflects the individual's responsibility for competence in practice. The ADA Code of Ethics Task Force reviewed and revised the 1999 Code of Ethics in March 2009, and the ADA Board of Directors, the CDR, and the House of Delegates approved it in May 2009. The 2009 Code of Ethics was published in the August 2009 *Journal of the American Dietetic Association* (pp. 1461–1467). The 2009 Code is in effect as of January 1, 2010, and the 1999 version of the code is no longer valid.[21]

The new code of ethics (see **Figure 7-2**) outlines ethics considerations in four areas: (1) responsibilities to the public, (2) responsibilities to clients, (3) responsibilities to the profession, and (4) responsibilities to colleagues and other professionals. Although the Code applies to all RDs and DTRs, discussing ethics in different practice settings helps dietetics practitioners to conceptualize ethical dilemmas they may face in their own practice.

The Code of Ethics also outlines the process for consideration of ethics issues and how ethics cases are handled. Disciplinary actions may be taken against a dietetics practitioner who is found to be in violation of the Code of Ethics. Disciplinary actions may include censure, probation, suspension of Academy membership, suspension of registration, expulsion from membership, or revocation of registration status.[22]

PREAMBLE

The Academy of Nutrition and Dietetics and its credentialing agency, the Commission on Dietetic Registration (CDR), believe it is in the best interest of the profession and the public it serves to have a Code of Ethics in place that provides guidance to dietetics practitioners in their professional practice and conduct. Dietetics practitioners have voluntarily adopted this Code of Ethics to reflect the values and ethical principles guiding the dietetics profession and to set forth commitments and obligations of the dietetics practitioner to the *public, clients, the profession, colleagues, and other professionals*. The current Code of Ethics was approved on June 2, 2009, by the ADA Board of Directors, House of Delegates, and the Commission on Dietetic Registration.

APPLICATION

The Code of Ethics applies to the following practitioners: (a) In its entirety to members of the Academy who are Registered Dietitians (RDs) or Dietetic Technicians, Registered (DTRs); (b) Except for sections dealing solely with the credential, to all members of the Academy who are not RDs or DTRs; and (c) Except for aspects dealing solely with membership, to all RDs and DTRs who are not members of the Academy. All individuals to whom the Code applies are referred to as "dietetics practitioners," and all such individuals who are RDs and DTRs shall be known as "credentialed practitioners." By accepting membership in to the Academy and/or accepting and maintaining CDR credentials, all members of the Academy and credentialed dietetics practitioners agree to abide by the Code.

PRINCIPLES

Fundamental Principles

1. The dietetics practitioner conducts himself/herself with honesty, integrity, and fairness.
2. The dietetics practitioner supports and promotes high standards of professional practice. The dietetics practitioner accepts the obligation to protect clients, the public, and the profession by upholding the Code of Ethics for the Profession of Dietetics and by reporting perceived violations of the Code through the processes established by the Academy and its credentialing agency, CDR.

Responsibilities to the Public

3. The dietetics practitioner considers the health, safety, and welfare of the public at all times.
   The dietetics practitioner will report inappropriate behavior or treatment of a client by another dietetics practitioner or other professionals.
4. The dietetics practitioner complies with all laws and regulations applicable or related to the profession or to the practitioner's ethical obligations as described in this Code.
   a. The dietetics practitioner must not be convicted of a crime under the laws of the United States, whether a felony or a misdemeanor, an essential element of which is dishonesty.
   b. The dietetics practitioner must not be disciplined by a state for conduct that would violate one or more of these principles.
   c. The dietetics practitioner must not commit an act of misfeasance or malfeasance that is directly related to the practice of the profession as determined by a court of competent jurisdiction, a licensing board, or an agency of a governmental body.

FIGURE 7–2 Academy of Nutrition and Dietetics Code of Ethics. *(continues)*
Courtesy of Commission on Dietetic Registration, Academy of Nutrition and Dietetics, Chicago, IL

5. The dietetics practitioner provides professional services with objectivity and with respect for the unique needs and values of individuals.
   a. The dietetics practitioner does not, in professional practice, discriminate against others on the basis of race, ethnicity, creed, religion, disability, gender, age, gender identity, sexual orientation, national origin, economic status, or any other legally protected category.
   b. The dietetics practitioner provides services in a manner that is sensitive to cultural differences.
   c. The dietetics practitioner does not engage in sexual harassment in connection with professional practice.
6. The dietetics practitioner does not engage in false or misleading practices or communications.
   a. The dietetics practitioner does not engage in false or deceptive advertising of his or her services.
   b. The dietetics practitioner promotes or endorses specific goods or products only in a manner that is not false and misleading.
   c. The dietetics practitioner provides accurate and truthful information in communicating with the public.
7. The dietetics practitioner withdraws from professional practice when unable to fulfill his or her professional duties and responsibilities to clients and others.
   a. The dietetics practitioner withdraws from practice when he/she has engaged in abuse of a substance such that it could affect his or her practice.
   b. The dietetics practitioner ceases practice when he or she has been adjudged by a court to be mentally incompetent.
   c. The dietetics practitioner will not engage in practice when he or she has a condition that substantially impairs his or her ability to provide effective service to others.

Responsibilities to Clients

8. The dietetics practitioner recognizes and exercises professional judgment within the limits of his or her qualifications and collaborates with others, seeks counsel, or makes referrals as appropriate.
9. The dietetics practitioner treats clients and patients with respect and consideration.
   a. The dietetics practitioner provides sufficient information to enable clients and others to make their own informed decisions.
   b. The dietetics practitioner respects the client's right to make decisions regarding the recommended plan of care, including consent, modification, or refusal.
10. The dietetics practitioner protects confidential information and makes full disclosure about any limitations on his or her ability to guarantee full confidentiality.
11. The dietetics practitioner, in dealing with and providing services to clients and others, complies with the same principles set forth above in "Responsibilities to the Public" (Principles #3–7).

Responsibilities to the Profession

12. The dietetics practitioner practices dietetics based on evidence-based principles and current information.
13. The dietetics practitioner presents reliable and substantiated information and interprets controversial information without personal bias, recognizing that legitimate differences of opinion exist.

FIGURE 7–2 Academy of Nutrition and Dietetics Code of Ethics. *(continued)*
Courtesy of Commission on Dietetic Registration, Academy of Nutrition and Dietetics, Chicago, IL

14. The dietetics practitioner assumes a life-long responsibility and accountability for personal competence in practice, consistent with accepted professional standards, continually striving to increase professional knowledge and skills and to apply them in practice.
15. The dietetics practitioner is alert to the occurrence of a real or potential conflict of interest and takes appropriate action whenever a conflict arises.
    a. The dietetics practitioner makes full disclosure of any real or perceived conflict of interest.
    b. When a conflict of interest cannot be resolved by disclosure, the dietetics practitioner takes such other action as may be necessary to eliminate the conflict, including recusal from an office, position, or practice situation.
16. The dietetics practitioner permits the use of his or her name for the purpose of certifying that dietetics services have been rendered only if he or she has provided or supervised the provision of those services.
17. The dietetics practitioner accurately presents professional qualifications and credentials.
    a. The dietetics practitioner, in seeking, maintaining, and using credentials provided by CDR, provides accurate information and complies with all requirements imposed by CDR. The dietetics practitioner uses CDR-awarded credentials ("RD" or "Registered Dietitian"; "DTR" or "Dietetic Technician, Registered"; "CS" or "Certified Specialist"; and "FADA" or "Fellow of the American Dietetic Association") only when the credential is current and authorized by CDR.
    b. The dietetics practitioner does not aid any other person in violating any CDR requirements, or in representing him or herself as CDR-credentialed when he or she is not.
18. The dietetics practitioner does not invite, accept, or offer gifts, monetary incentives, or other considerations that affect or reasonably give an appearance of affecting his/her professional judgment.

Clarification of Principle:

a. Whether a gift, incentive, or other item of consideration shall be viewed to affect, or give the appearance of affecting, a dietetics practitioner's professional judgment is dependent on all factors relating to the transaction, including the amount or value of the consideration, the likelihood that the practitioner's judgment will or is intended to be affected, the position held by the practitioner, and whether the consideration is offered or generally available to persons other than the practitioner.
b. It shall not be a violation of this principle for a dietetic compensation as a consultant or employee or as part of a research grant or corporate sponsorship program, provided the relationship is openly disclosed and the practitioner acts with integrity in performing the services or responsibilities.
c. This principle shall not preclude a dietetics practitioner from accepting gifts of nominal value, attendance at educational programs, meals in connection with educational exchanges of information, free samples of products, or similar items, as long as such items are not offered in exchange for or with the expectation of, and do not result in, conduct or services that are contrary to the practitioner's professional judgment.

FIGURE 7–2 Academy of Nutrition and Dietetics Code of Ethics. *(continued)*
Courtesy of Commission on Dietetic Registration, Academy of Nutrition and Dietetics, Chicago, IL

> d. The test for appearance of impropriety is whether the conduct would create in reasonable minds a perception that the dietetics practitioner's ability to carry out professional responsibilities with integrity, impartiality, and competence is impaired.
>
> ## Responsibilities to Colleagues and Other Professionals
> 19. The dietetics practitioner demonstrates respect for the values, rights, knowledge, and skills of colleagues and other professionals.
>   a. The dietetics practitioner does not engage in dishonest, misleading, or inappropriate business practices that demonstrate a disregard for the rights or interests of others.
>   b. The dietetics practitioner provides objective evaluations of performance for employees and coworkers, candidates for employment, students, professional association memberships, awards, or scholarships, making all reasonable efforts to avoid bias in the professional evaluation of others.

FIGURE 7–2 Academy of Nutrition and Dietetics Code of Ethics. *(continued)*
Courtesy of Commission on Dietetic Registration, Academy of Nutrition and Dietetics, Chicago, IL

The Code of Ethics section of the Academy website (www.eatright.org) offers a wealth of information about the Code and its applications. The site includes numerous educational resource links as well as a "Watch and Learn" video presentation about the Code and why it is important to dietetics professionals and the profession of dietetics.

Summary

Each dietetic student should have the goal of becoming a credentialed dietetics practitioner. Although completion of an associate or baccalaureate degree in dietetics is a worthy achievement, earning the professional credential of DTR or RD opens the doors for successful professional practice. This credential is your clients' assurance of your qualifications to practice, and it indicates that you actively work to update yourself on the latest information about food and nutrition issues. Licensure indicates that the state in which you practice recognizes your professional competence and expertise.

Specialty certification will become more common in the years ahead, as dietetics practice becomes increasingly complex and diverse. Professional credentialing is the mark of quality practice; it assures the public that the dietetic technician or registered dietitian is providing the highest quality in dietetics services.

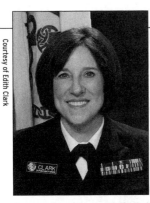

Courtesy of Edith Clark

Profile of a Professional

Captain Edith Clark, MBA, RD, CDE

Chief Dietitian Officer for the Commissioned Corps of the U.S. Public Health Service

Director, Nutrition Services at Phoenix Indian Medical
  Center

Director, Southwestern Dietetic Internship Consortium

Education:

BS in Foods and Nutrition, Montana State University,
  Bozeman, Montana

MBA, The University of Phoenix

Do you have any other professional credentials?

Certified Diabetes Educator (CDE), National Certification Board for Diabetes Educators
ServSafe Certification, The National Restaurant Association Educational Foundation
Certificate of Training in Adult Weight Management, Commission on Dietetic
  Registration, The Academy of Nutrition and Dietetics

How did you first learn about dietetics as a profession?

I learned about dietetics when I first started my undergraduate program at Montana
State. However, I did not decide to become a Registered Dietitian until the end of my
second year of college.

What was your route to registration as a dietitian?

I completed the Didactic Program in Dietetics at Montana State and then was
matched to the Dietetic Internship at Milwaukee County Medical Complex in
Milwaukee, Wisconsin.

Describe your career path thus far.

I have worked as a foodservice director for a state hospital, a rural community
hospital, and a large private city hospital. I am now director of nutrition services for
a 127-bed Indian Health Service hospital in Phoenix, Arizona. This facility provides
full-time inpatient nutrition services, full-time outpatient nutrition services, and a
full-time foodservice staff on site for patients and employee meals. In addition, we
provide nutrition services to six outlying Native American communities. Some of
these services are provided to patients one-on-one in a clinic setting, while others are
public health and community-based programs. Examples of this are nutrition programs for participants in the preschool program and after-school programs and a
community garden project with elders and youth working side-by-side in an effort to
have access to healthy vegetables.

  I am also the program director of the Southwestern Dietetic Internship Consortium.
This is a program that was approved in 2005 with a focus on American Indian/Alaska
Native nutrition. Every one of our interns has been from a federally recognized Native
American tribe.

  I am the Chief Dietitian Officer for the Commissioned Corps of the U.S. Public
Health Service. In this role, one of the responsibilities is to support the agenda of the
Office of the Surgeon General. I also represent the nearly 100 RDs who are commis-
sioned officers in the U.S. Public Health Service.

What are some examples of your professional involvement?

I am a member of the Academy of Nutrition and Dietetics as well as the local and
state dietetics associations. I'm also actively involved in the Commissioned Officers
Association, which deals with issues affecting dietitians in the commission corps as
well as on all officers.

Have you received honors or awards?

I have received a variety of awards through the Commissioned Corps of the U.S. Public
Health Service and have received two Indian Health Service National Director's Awards.

How is teamwork important to you in your position?

Teamwork is critical in any position. This has been especially true in my role as a department director, and also as a provider of medical nutrition therapy and other roles filled by RDs. Dietitians are also excellent candidates to be considered for case manager positions, which rely heavily on teamwork.

I've been involved in several team projects at the national level with the Indian Health Service, including developing a standardized curriculum for diabetes education and developing a standardized curriculum for patients with gestational diabetes. One of the major team efforts was the development of the Southwestern Dietetic Internship Consortium. It is the only dietetic internship designed to prepare dietetics professionals to work in Native American communities. Seeing this project brought to fruition with its approval in November 2005 was most gratifying.

What excites you about dietetics and the future of our profession?

I think this is a fabulous time to be a dietitian! There are many varied opportunities for dietetics professionals. Some of these opportunities are in traditional roles, but many are evolving in nontraditional areas. There are many great opportunities to work in federal agencies. You can find more about dietitian positions with the Indian Health Service at www.ihs.gov. This is also a great time to explore job opportunities as an officer in the Commissioned Corps of the U.S. Public Health Service. You can find more about what it means to be a commissioned corps officer at www.usphs.gov.

What words of wisdom do you have for future dietetics professionals?

Study hard during your undergraduate program and keep your eyes on your science and math courses. These lay the foundation for your future. Also, take time to volunteer your time as a diet aide in a hospital or nursing home to learn more about applications of medical nutrition therapy.

Suggested Activities

1. Talk to someone who has recently taken the registration examination for RDs or DTRs. What was his or her reaction to the experience? What suggestions does he or she have for preparing for the exam?

2. Look in the back of the *Journal of the Academy of Nutrition and Dietetics* or go online and look at the RD exam review ads. What kinds of tools are available to help you prepare for the test? How much do they cost? What are some less expensive ways you could prepare for the credentialing exam?

3. Who is your state continuing education coordinator? If possible, talk to this person and find out what kinds of continuing education events he or she approves. What process must be followed to get an event approved for continuing education credit?

4. Attend a continuing education event with a dietetics professional, faculty member, or another student. What kind of documentation must be provided for an attendee to receive continuing education credits?

5. Find out if your state has licensure for dietitians. If so, work with your teacher to invite someone to your class to talk about licensure, what it means in your state, and how it was obtained in the legislature. What is the process for becoming licensed in your state?

6. Pick another professional credential besides the DTR or RD that you might be interested in pursuing. Visit the website of the certifying agency and find out exactly what you would need to do to earn that credential or certification.

7. Talk with a dietetics professional about his or her career portfolio. Ask the professional to share with you what it was like to do self-assessment to determine continuing education goals. What kinds of continuing education opportunities has this person pursued to meet professional development goals?

8. What kind of continuing education requirements are there for other professional credentials? How do these requirements compare with dietetics requirements?

Selected Websites

- www.diabeteseducator.org—American Association of Diabetes Educators; offers information on the Board Certified in Advanced Diabetes Management (BC-ADM) credential.
- www.acsm.org—American College of Sports Medicine (ACSM); offers information on the various ACSM credentials.
- www.acefitness.org—American Council on Exercise (ACE); provides information on the various ACE credentials.
- www.eatright.org—Academy of Nutrition and Dietetics site offers purchase information for the *CDR RD Exam Study Guide* and the *CDR DTR Exam Study Guide.*
- www.cdrnet.org—CDR site offers information about CDR specialty credentials.
- www.dietitianexam.com—DietitianExam.com review program.
- www.iaacn.org—International and American Associations of Clinical Nutritionists; offers information on the Certified Clinical Nutritionist (CCN) credential.
- www.nafem.org—North American Association of Food Equipment Manufacturers; offers information on the Certified Foodservice Professional (CFSP) credential.
- www.ncbde.org—National Certification Board for Diabetes Educators; offers information on the Certified Diabetes Educator (CDE) credential.
- www.rdinaflash.com—"RD in a Flash" flash cards.

References

1. *Webster's New Universal Unabridged Dictionary.* 2nd ed. New York: Simon & Schuster; 1983.
2. Commission on Dietetic Registration. Available at: http://www.cdrnet.org/about/index .cfm. Accessed May 5, 2012.
3. Woodward NM. The past, present, and future of dietetics credentialing. Future Search Conference: Challenging the Future of Dietetic Education and Credentialing. Background Papers. Chicago: The American Dietetic Association and the Commission on Dietetic Registration, June 12–14, 1994.

4. Commission on Dietetic Registration. Available at http://www.cdrnet.org/PDFs /Setting%20the%20Standards%20since%201969website.pdf. Accessed May 18, 2012.

5. Commission on Dietetic Registration. Available at http://www.cdrnet.org/PDFs /Setting%20the%20Standards%20since%201969website.pdf. Accessed May 18, 2012.

6. Breeding & Associates Educational Resource Center. Available at: http://www .dietitianworkshops.com/. Accessed May 5, 2012.

7. Inman Seminars. Available at: http://www.inmanassoc.com. Accessed May 5, 2012.

8. RD in a Flash. Available at: http://www.rdinaflash.com. Accessed May 5, 2012.

9. DietitianExam.com. Available at: http://www.dietitianexam.com. Accessed May 5, 2012.

10. Commission on Dietetic Registration. Professional Development Portfolio Guide. Available at: http://www.cdrnet.org/pdrcenter. Accessed May 5, 2012.

11. Commission on Dietetic Registration. Specialty Certifications. Available at: http://www .cdrnet.org/certifications. Accessed May 5, 2012.

12. Commission on Dietetic Registration. Setting the Standards Since 1969. Available at: http://www.cdrnet.org/PDFs/Setting%20the%20Standards%20since%201969website .pdf. Accessed May 18, 2012.

13. Commission on Dietetic Registration. Fellow of the Academy of Nutrition and Dietetics. Available at: http://www.cdrnet.org/certifications/fellows/fmap.cfm. Accessed May 18, 2012.

14. American Dietetic Association. Final Report of the Phase 2 Future Practice & Education Task Force. Available at: http://www.cdrnet.org/pdfs/Final%20Task%20Force%20 Report%20July%2015%2008%20FINAL.pdf. Accessed January 31, 2010.

15. Commission on Dietetic Registration. State Licensure. Available at: http://www.cdrnet .org/certifications. Accessed May 5, 2012.

16. Commission on Dietetic Registration. State Licensure Agency List. Available at: http:// www.cdrnet.org/certifications/licensure/agencylist.cfm. Accessed May 5, 2012.

17. Academy of Nutrition and Dietetics. Evidence-Based Practice: Definition-Description and Key Considerations. Available at: http://www.eatright.org/Members/content .aspx?id=8333. Accessed May 5, 2012.

18. Evidence Analysis Library. Available at: http://www.adaevidencelibrary.com/default .cfm?auth=1. Accessed May 5, 2012.

19. Academy of Nutrition and Dietetics. Dietetics Practice-Based Research Network. Available at: http://www.eatright.org/Members/content.aspx?id=8336. Accessed May 5, 2012.

20. Academy of Nutrition and Dietetics. Practice Tips. Standards of Practice and Professional Performance. Available at: http://www.eatright.org/sop/. Accessed January 31, 2010.

21. Academy of Nutrition and Dietetics. The Code of Ethics. Available at: http://www .eatright.org/codeofethics/. Accessed May 5, 2012.

22. American Dietetic Association/Commission on Dietetic Registration Code of Ethics for the Profession of Dietetics and Process for Consideration of Ethics Issues. *J Am Diet Assoc.* 2009;109:1461–1467.

Professional Organizations

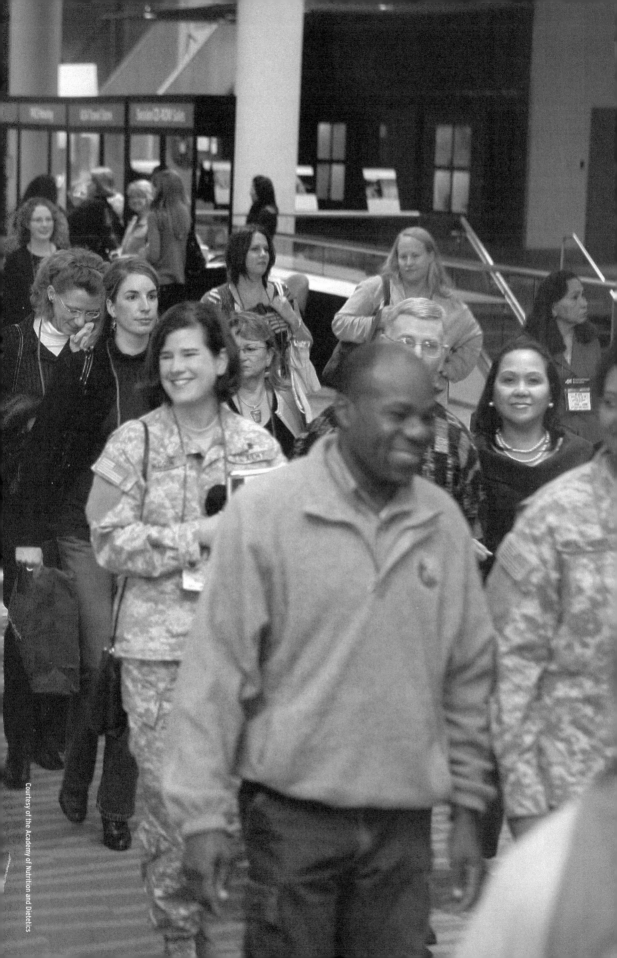

Why Join a Professional Association?

The benefits of membership in a professional association are numerous for those already practicing in the field and for students who aspire to be practicing professionals. Most professional associations offer student membership and provide resources for educational preparation and career building. Specific benefits of student membership include networking with other students in the field; leadership experiences; eligibility for scholarships and awards; access to the latest in online and print media in the field; access to job opportunities; reduced rates at conferences; and special rates on credit cards, car rentals, and hotels.

The Academy of Nutrition and Dietetics

The Academy of Nutrition and Dietetics is the largest association of food and nutrition professionals in the world.[1] Founded in Cleveland, Ohio, in 1917, as the American Dietetic Association, the Academy has grown to almost 72,000 members.[2] The purpose of this chapter is to help you understand the mission, vision, and values of the Academy of Nutrition and Dietetics and to become knowledgeable about its structure and organization. Other professional associations that may be of interest to dietetics professionals are also introduced.

Who Are the Members of the Academy of Nutrition and Dietetics?

The Academy of Nutrition and Dietetics offers five membership classifications: student, active, retired, international, and honorary.[3] You may utilize several of these membership categories as you move through your professional life.

The **student member** category is open to anyone who meets one of the following criteria:

- Is a student enrolled in an ACEND-accredited dietetics program or supervised practice program who does not meet requirements for active membership, or
- Is a student enrolled in a regionally accredited, postsecondary education program that is non-ACEND accredited (this classification is available to students who state their intent to enter an ACEND-accredited program), or
- Is a current active member returning to school on a full-time basis to complete a baccalaureate or advanced degree or to complete an ACEND-accredited supervised practice program (DI or CP). Annual verification is required for this category.

The student membership has a 6-year time limit. The current dues are $50/year.

An **active member** can be any person who has earned the appropriate degree, meets the academic requirements specified by ACEND, and meets one or more of the following criteria:

- Is an RD, a DTR, or has established eligibility to write the registration examination for dietitians or dietetic technicians administered by the CDR.
- Has completed a baccalaureate degree or a supervised practice program (DI, CP, or AP4 program) accredited by ACEND.
- Is an active member in Dietitians of Canada.
- Has earned either a master's or doctoral degree and holds one degree (baccalaureate, master's, or doctoral) in one of the following areas: dietetics, food and nutrition, nutrition, community or public health nutrition, food science, or foodservice systems management.
- Has completed an ACEND-approved associate degree program for dietetic technicians.

Retired member status can be held by any current active member who is:

- At least 62 years of age and no longer employed in dietetics practice or education, or
- Retired on total (permanent) disability.

See your dietetics program director for student member information or call the Academy of Nutrition and Dietetics at 1-800-877-1600. Alternatively, you can visit the Academy website (www.eatright.org) for membership information. Joining the Academy of Nutrition and Dietetics as a student is an excellent way to learn about the dietetics profession and become familiar with its publications, activities, and other benefits (**Figure 8–1**).

The **international member** category includes any person who has completed formal training in food, nutrition, or dietetics outside the United States and U.S. territories. Membership in this category requires verification from the country's professional dietetic association or regulatory body.

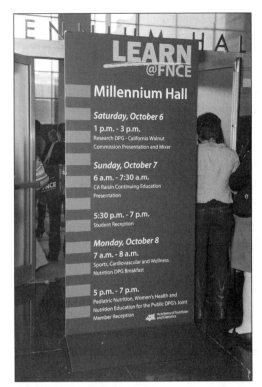

FIGURE 8–1 The Food and Nutrition Conference and Expo (FNCE), the annual meeting of the Academy of Nutrition and Dietetics, offers networking opportunities for students.
Courtesy of the Academy of Nutrition and Dietetics

Finally, the **honorary member** category is a special honor awarded to an individual who has made a notable contribution to the field of nutrition and dietetics and has been invited to be an honorary member by the Academy of Nutrition and Dietetics's Board of Directors.[4]

Mission, Vision, Philosophy, and Values

In 2008 (when it was still the ADA), the Academy of Nutrition and Dietetics Board of Directors endorsed a strategic plan that lays out goals based on the Academy of Nutrition and Dietetics's vision, mission, and values. The plan is reviewed and updated regularly to represent the philosophical base of the Academy.

The Academy of Nutrition and Dietetics' vision statement is "Optimize the nation's health through food and nutrition."[5] The Academy's vision statement helps members understand the role the Academy hopes to assume in the future.

The Academy's mission statement is "Empower members to be the nation's food and nutrition leaders."[5]

The Academy's values serve as a guide to action and a statement of attributes toward which all dietitians should strive. The Academy's values are:

- Customer focus—meet the needs and exceed the expectations of all customers
- Integrity—act ethically with accountability for lifelong learning and commitment to excellence
- Innovation—embrace change with creativity and strategic thinking
- Social responsibility—make decisions with consideration for inclusivity as well as environmental, economic, and social implications[5]

Finally, the 3 strategic goals and 16 strategies of the Academy of Nutrition and Dietetics that act to guide it in its activities are:

Goal 1: The public trusts and chooses registered dietitians as food and nutrition experts.

- Create a respected brand.
- Establish value to the public through effective programs, services, and initiatives offered to registered dietitians.
- Take proactive positions based on evidence.
- Work cooperatively with the international dietetics community.

Goal 2: The Academy improves the health of Americans.

- Impact food and nutrition policies.
- Provide opportunities for members to participate in the legislative and regulatory processes at local, state, and federal levels.
- Strengthen relationships with external organizations to further Academy initiatives.
- Inform the public about ways to improve its health.
- Equip members to use research in their work.
- Strengthen cultural competence to address health disparities.

Goal 3: Members and prospective members view the Academy of Nutrition and Dietetics as key to professional success.

- Ensure competence through education, accreditation, and certification.
- Provide state-of-the-art professional development opportunities for career success.
- Provide relevant and valued products and services for diverse member audiences.
- Provide leadership opportunities to enhance knowledge and skills for success in practice, workplace, and communities.
- Provide research and resources that can be translated into evidence-based practice.
- Attract members from underrepresented groups.[5]

Academy of Nutrition and Dietetics Headquarters

The Academy of Nutrition and Dietetics' headquarters are located in Chicago, Illinois. It houses the paid staff members who carry on the Academy's day-to-day business. These employees work in assigned groups that serve to support different aspects of the Academy of Nutrition and Dietetics' focus.

Also located in the same Chicago location are the Academy of Nutrition and Dietetics Foundation and the offices of the Commission on Dietetic Registration (CDR).

The Foundation funds education initiatives that promote public nutrition, health, and well-being. The Foundation is a nonprofit corporation and is the largest private grantor of scholarship and fellowship funds in the field of dietetics. Students in dietetics and related fields are encouraged to apply for Foundation scholarships. Applications are typically due the middle of February each year, with awards made for the following academic year. Dietetic education program directors receive information about these scholarships every fall.[6]

The CDR is the credentialing arm of the Academy of Nutrition and Dietetics. The CDR credentials individuals who have met its standards for competency to practice in the profession. The function of the CDR is discussed in Chapter 7.[7]

The Academy also retains paid employees at an office in Washington, DC. These employees work on the Academy's behalf on legislative matters that affect the future of the dietetics profession. Members may call the Academy of Nutrition and Dietetics Government Relations office in Washington, DC, at 1-800-877-0877 with questions about legislative activities or issues affecting dietetics at the state or federal level (**Figure 8–2**).[8]

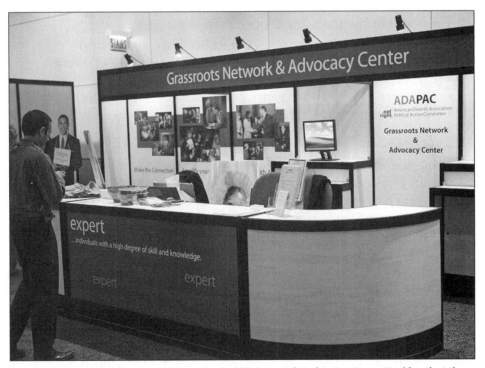

FIGURE 8–2 The ANDPAC (Academy of Nutrition and Dietetics Political Action Committee) booth at the Food and Nutrition Conference and Expo.
Courtesy of the Academy of Nutrition and Dietetics

The Volunteer Element of the Academy of Nutrition and Dietetics

The officers of the Academy are volunteers who are elected by the membership. Major offices are elected by national ballot; members of particular subgroups, such as Dietetic Practice Groups, elect their own officers.

The work of the Academy is accomplished by two major entities: the Board of Directors and the House of Delegates.

The Board of Directors

The Academy of Nutrition and Dietetics is governed by a Board of Directors.[9] In this role, the Board of Directors does the following:

- Sets and monitors strategic direction
- Oversees fiscal planning
- Provides leadership for professional initiatives
- Selects, supports, and assesses the chief executive officer and conducts an annual performance appraisal
- Appoints persons to represent the Academy
- Establishes guidelines and policies for appeals, publications, awards, and honors
- Administers and enforces the professional Code of Ethics in conjunction with the CDR and the House of Delegates
- Exercises such powers and performs all lawful acts permitted or required under the Illinois Not-for-Profit Corporation Act

The Board of Directors has 18 members:

- President, elected by the general membership (1-year term)
- President-Elect, elected by the general membership (1-year term)
- Past-President (l-year term)
- Treasurer, elected by the general membership (2-year term)
- Three Directors at Large, elected by the general membership (3-year term)
- Speaker of the House of Delegates
- Speaker-Elect of the House of Delegates
- Four House of Delegates Directors, elected by the House of Delegates (2-year term)
- One Young Member
- Two Public Members, appointed by the Board of Directors (2-year term)
- Academy of Nutrition and Dietetics Foundation Chair, elected by the Foundation (1-year term)
- Academy of Nutrition and Dietetics CEO (nonvoting)

The House of Delegates

The Academy of Nutrition and Dietetics House of Delegates (HOD) is the deliberative body of the Academy, acting as the voice of Academy members.[10] The House of Delegates governs the profession and develops policy on major professional issues. In its role of governing the profession, the House of Delegates does the following:

- Monitors and evaluates trends affecting the profession
- Monitors member issues and mega issues, and the resulting actions
- Reviews, debates, and approves professional standards, including standards of education and practice
- Adopts and revises with the CDR a Code of Ethics for dietetics practitioners, disciplinary procedures for unethical conduct, and reinstatement conditions
- Provides direction for quality management in dietetics practice
- Identifies and develops position statements
- Assists with recruitment and retention efforts related to leadership development
- Serves as the voice of the members of the profession

The Academy of Nutrition and Dietetics House of Delegates has 100 members:

- 66 Affiliate Delegates—elected by the affiliate members and representing the 53 affiliate dietetic associations
- 18 Professional Issues Delegates—representing the 29 dietetic practice groups and are elected by the general Academy membership
- 10 At-Large Delegates—one delegate representing ACEND, one delegate representing CDR, one delegate representing student members, two delegates representing DTRs, one delegate representing retired members, one delegate representing members under 30 years of age, and three delegates-at-large representing the broad membership
- 6 House of Delegates Directors—comprising the House of Delegates Leadership Team, who are also members of the Academy of Nutrition and Dietetics Board of Directors

The full membership of the House of Delegates meets twice a year, immediately before the start of the Food and Nutrition Conference and Expo each fall (**Figure 8–3**) and at the House of Delegates Mid-Year Meeting; typically held at the end of April or beginning of May. Because delegates are the elected representatives of the Academy of Nutrition and Dietetics members in their respective states, they bring to these HOD meetings the views of their constituents back home. Observers are welcome to attend any of these sessions to gain a fuller appreciation of how the work of the Academy is carried out. The formal House of Delegates meeting, during which agenda items are voted on, is held on Sunday each time the House of Delegates meets. It is a formal and impressive event.

State Affiliates and District Dietetic Associations

Each state plus the District of Columbia has its own state dietetic association affiliated with the Academy of Nutrition and Dietetics.

When an individual joins the Academy of Nutrition and Dietetics, a percentage of his or her dues is rebated to the state dietetic association with which he or she wishes to affiliate. Although most individuals are members of the affiliate dietetic association of the state in which they live or work, a 1998 bylaws amendment now allows individuals the option to designate

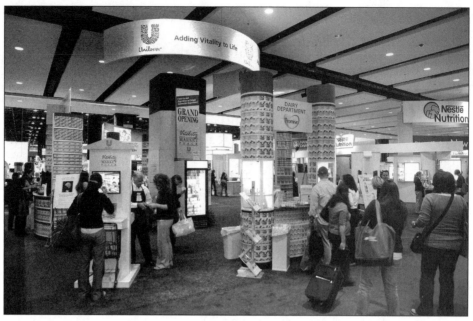

FIGURE 8–3 The exhibit hall at the Food and Nutrition Conference and Expo.
Courtesy of the Academy of Nutrition and Dietetics

any state dietetic association for their membership. State dietetic associations elect their own officers and host their own meetings once or twice a year.[11]

Each state association is made up of district dietetic associations that serve the needs of dietitians in specific geographic areas within the state. Currently, there are approximately 230 district associations in the United States. District associations may cover a single metropolitan area or several counties. Membership in district associations is not automatic. These groups receive no rebates from the national level and typically charge a separate membership fee to support their programming efforts.

Involvement in district and state dietetic associations is a great way for new dietetics graduates to become involved in a professional organization. Opportunities for leadership development and personal/professional growth abound in these groups.

Dietetic Practice Groups

Dietetic Practice Groups (DPGs) are composed of individuals who have a common interest in a particular area of dietetics practice, regardless of membership classification or employment status. Anyone with an interest in the particular area of practice can join a DPG, and you can join as many DPGs as desired. A DPG may be formed when at least 300 members petition the House of Delegates Council on Professional Issues to form such a group.

DPGs are national in scope and have their own elected officers and dues. These groups engage in activities that meet the needs of their members, such as producing newsletters or providing continuing education events. They also provide members with the opportunity to develop leadership skills through participation on committees or through appointment or election to offices. See **Table 8–1** for a list of the 28 current DPGs of the Academy of Nutrition and Dietetics.[12]

TABLE 8–1

Academy of Nutrition and Dietetics Dietetic Practice Groups

Dietetic Practice Group	Focus
Behavioral Health Nutrition	Mission is "to impact the nutrition of the behavioral health populations we serve."
Clinical Nutrition Management	Managers who direct clinical nutrition programs across the continuum of care.
Diabetes Care and Education	Members involved in patient education and professional education as well as research for the management of diabetes mellitus.
Nutrition and Dietetic Educators and Preceptors	Educators and preceptors of nutrition and dietetics practitioners for entry and advanced levels of nutrition and dietetics practice.
Dietetic Technicians in Practice	DTRs, dietetic technician educators, and others who are interested in DTR practice and issues that directly affect the DTR
Dietetics in Heath Care Communities	Practitioners typically employed under contract who provide nutrition consultation to acute and long-term-care facilities, home care companies, healthcare agencies, and the foodservice industry.
Dietitians in Business and Communications	Food and nutrition professionals who are working with local or global corporations,businesses, or organizations in food, nutrition, communications, public relations, and healthcare industries, or who are self-employed or business owners.
Dietitians in Nutrition Support	Dietitians who integrate the science of enteral and parenteral nutrition in order to provide appropriate nutrition support therapy to individuals encompassing adults, pediatrics, inpatients, outpatients, home care, and transplantation.
Food and Culinary Professionals	Members who promote food education and culinary skills to enhance quality of life and health of the public.
Healthy Aging	Practitioners who provide and manage nutrition programs and services to older adults in a variety of settings—community, home, healthcare facilities, and education and research facilities.
Hunger and Environmental Nutrition	Members optimize the nation's health by promoting access to nutritious food and clean water from a secure and sustainable food system.
Infectious Diseases Nutrition	Dietetics professionals sharing cutting-edge information on nutrition management of infectious diseases and providing an avenue for research, monitoring, and advocacy for nutrition intervention.
Management in Food and Nutrition Systems	Food and nutrition care managers generally employed in institutions, colleges, and universities, and includes directors of department of facilities, administrative dietitians, and technicians.

(continues)

TABLE 8–1

Academy of Nutrition and Dietetics Dietetic Practice Groups (*continued*)

Dietetic Practice Group	Focus
Medical Nutrition Practice Group	Mission is to empower members to be the recognized leaders who provide exemplary nutrition care.
Nutrition Education for the Public	Practitioners involved in the design, implementation, and evaluation of nutrition education programs for target populations.
Nutrition Educators of Health Professionals	Members involved in education and communication with physicians, nurses, dentists, and other healthcare professionals.
Nutrition Entrepreneurs	Members are shaping the future of dietetics by pursuing innovative and creative ways of providing nutrition products and services to consumers, industry, media, and businesses.
Nutrition in Complementary Care	Dietetics professionals interested in the study of alternative and complementary therapies.
Oncology Nutrition	Nutrition professionals involved in the care of cancer patients, cancer prevention, and research.
Pediatric Nutrition	Practitioners who provide nutrition services for the pediatric population in a wide variety of settings.
Public Health/Community Nutrition	Nutrition professionals who provide nutrition services to all age groups in a community setting.
Renal Dietitians	Focuses on chronic kidney disease and provides educational materials and resources for both professionals and patients/clients.
Research	Members propose, assist with, complete, manage, and disseminate research projects conducted in clinical, community, healthcare, laboratory, and academic settings.
School Nutrition Services	School foodservice directors and nutrition educators employed in child nutrition programs and corporate dietitians working in companies supplying products or services to school foodservice operations.
Sports, Cardiovascular, and Wellness Nutritionists	Nutrition professionals with expertise in promoting healthy, active lifestyles through excellence in nutrition for sports performance, cardiovascular health, wellness, and the prevention and treatment of disordered eating.
Vegetarian Nutrition	Nutrition professionals in community, clinical, education, or foodservice settings who wish to learn about plant-based diets and provide support to individuals following a vegetarian lifestyle.
Weight Management	Supports the highest level of professional practice in the prevention and treatment of overweight and obesity throughout the life cycle.
Women's Health	Practitioners addressing women's health and nutrition care issues throughout the life cycle.

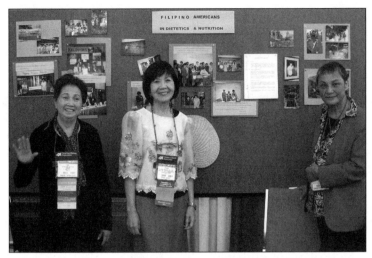

FIGURE 8–4 Members of the Filipino Americans in Dietetics and Nutrition at their booth at the Food and Nutrition Conference and Expo.
Courtesy of Bea Dykes, FADAN Member Interest Group

In addition to the DPGs, members may also choose to join a Member Interest Group (MIG). MIGs provide a way for members with common interests, issues, or backgrounds to connect. Unlike the affiliate, district, and DPG groups, the MIGs are not based on practice or geographic location. The current MIGs are:

- Chinese Americans in Dietetics and Nutrition
- Fifty Plus in Nutrition and Dietetics
- Filipino Americans in Dietetics and Nutrition (Figure 8–4)
- Latinos and Hispanics in Dietetics and Nutrition
- Muslims in Dietetics and Nutrition
- National Organization of Blacks in Dietetics and Nutrition
- National Organization of Men in Nutrition

Honors and Awards Bestowed by the Academy of Nutrition and Dietetics

Each year the Academy of Nutrition and Dietetics, the Academy of Nutrition and Dietetics Foundation, and DPGs honor individuals who have demonstrated outstanding contributions to the profession of dietetics. The **Marjorie Hulsizer Copher Award** is the highest honor the Academy can bestow on one of its members. Persons nominated for this honor must have contributed to the Academy of Nutrition and Dietetics through long, active participation and service. The recipient of this award is considered a trailblazer for the profession and someone who has contributed uniquely to the advancement of the profession and is a source of inspiration to other members. The Copher Award has been presented every year since 1945.[13]

The **Lenna Frances Cooper Memorial Lecturer** presents a major paper related to his or her work in dietetics. The presentation of this lecture is a highlight of each Food and Nutrition Conference and Exhibition of the Academy of Nutrition and Dietetics. The topic presented is one of widespread interest to Academy members and is normally associated with the lecturer's work. The recipient of this honor is a recognized speaker who has made noteworthy contributions to the profession of dietetics. There has been a Cooper Lecturer recognized every year at the Annual Meeting of the Academy since 1962.[14]

The **Academy of Nutrition and Dietetics Medallion** is awarded each year to a maximum of eight members of the Academy of Nutrition and Dietetics. Recipients of the Medallion Award are recognized for their exceptional service to the Academy and other food and nutrition associations, for professional leadership abilities, and for the fact that they have been instrumental in moving the profession of dietetics forward. They also have demonstrated personal characteristics of dedication to the high standards of the Academy of Nutrition and Dietetics, acting as a source of inspiration to others and exhibiting devotion to the spirit of service to others in dietetics, allied fields, and the community. The first Medallions were given in 1976 (**Figure 8–5**), and recipients of this award showcase the diversity of Academy members and their areas of practice.[15]

Honorary membership in the Academy of Nutrition and Dietetics is one of the highest awards given to nonmembers. Each honorary member brings honor to the Academy. Qualifications for nomination to honorary membership include distinguished contributions to dietetics through professional

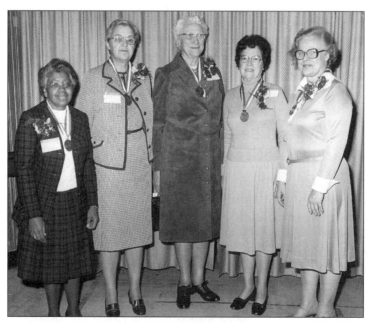

FIGURE 8–5 The first recipients of the Medallion Award. From left to right: Mildred Bunton, Grace Stumpf, Margaret Terrell, Ruby Linn, and Louise Irwin.
Courtesy of the Academy of Nutrition and Dietetics

knowledge, technical expertise, and promotion of the Academy of Nutrition and Dietetics' mission, vision, and values; demonstration of good will through notable national or international service to the advancement of the profession and/or the Academy; and promotion of dietetics professionals as contributors to the optimal health and nutritional status of the public.

The first honorary membership was awarded in 1954.[4]

The **Academy of Nutrition and Dietetics Foundation Awards for Excellence in Practice** showcases individuals who have demonstrated exceptional performance in a practice area of dietetics through innovation and creativity in practice. Six awards for excellence, representing the following areas of dietetics practice, are given each year: Community Dietetics, Clinical Nutrition, Consultation and Business Practice, Management Practice, Dietetic Education and Research, and Dietetic Technology.[16]

Among the many other awards administered by the Foundation that recognize and support dietetics professionals are the following:

- 12 Continuing Education Awards, ranging from $375 to $5,000 each
- 15 Recognition Awards, ranging from $300 to $25,000 each
- 5 International Awards, ranging from $1,000 to $25,000 each[16]

Some examples of these awards are:

- Allene Vaden Grant for Foodservice Management
- Anita Owen Recognition Award for Innovative Nutrition Education
- Judy Ford Stokes Award for Innovation in Administrative Dietetics
- PepsiCo Healthy Lifestyles Innovation Research Grant
- Mary Abbott Hess Award for Recognition of an Innovative Food/Culinary Effort[16]

In addition, during the past 5 years, the Academy of Nutrition and Dietetics Foundation has awarded 900 students with $1.4 million in scholarship money.[16]

Why Should I Become a Member of the Academy of Nutrition and Dietetics?

Membership in a professional association is a privilege. Professional associations such as the Academy of Nutrition and Dietetics provide opportunities for personal and professional growth, leadership, and lasting friendships. Whereas one dietitian alone may not feel that he or she can make a difference, the strength of almost 70,000 dietitians can make their voices heard in setting public policy or influencing public opinion. The Academy plays a key role in influencing issues such as healthcare reform, food labeling, child nutrition programs, nutrition screening for the elderly, and long-term care. The Academy provides expert testimony at congressional hearings and comments on proposed federal and state legislation. The Academy also publishes position papers, which outline the Academy of Nutrition and Dietetics's stand on a variety of timely, and sometimes controversial, topics. The Academy's website (www.eatright.org) has an extensive listing of member services and benefits.[17]

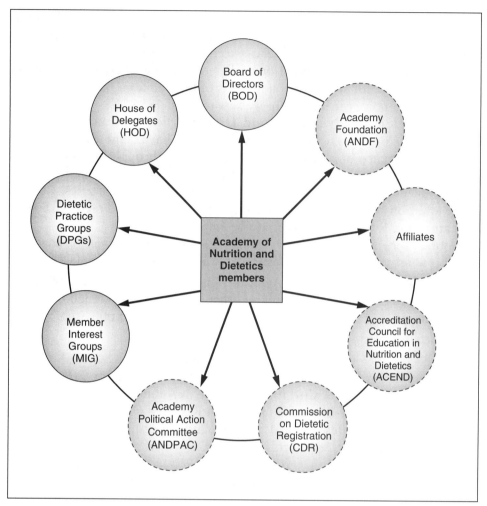

FIGURE 8–6 Academy of Nutrition and Dietetics Organization Units: Academy of Nutrition and Dietetics Foundation and Affiliates—legal autonomy; CDR and ACEND—administrative autonomy; AND-PAC—regulated by the Federal Elections Commission.
Courtesy of the Academy of Nutrition and Dietetics

The Academy of Nutrition and Dietetics also conducts a number of important programs, campaigns, and other outreach efforts to promote health and well-being and to position dietetics professionals as nutrition experts. A diagram of the Academy of Nutrition and Dietetics Organizational Units, previously discussed in this chapter, is shown in **Figure 8–6**.

Other Professional Associations

Dietetics professionals are often involved in numerous professional associations that may relate to their professional activities and interests. Each of these associations has its own mission, agenda, and member benefits. Most of these have a student membership category, which provides an excellent opportunity for students to gain valuable networking experience and resources for professional study and growth (**Table 8–2**).

TABLE 8–2

Selected Professional Associations

Organization	Address and Phone	Website Address	Publication(s) Available	Student Membership	Membership Dues
American Association of Family and Consumer Sciences (AAFCS)	400 N. Columbus Street, Suite 202 Alexandria, VA 22314 Phone: 703-706-4600	www.aafcs.org	*Journal of Family and Consumer Sciences*	Yes	$60
American College of Sports Medicine (ACSM)	401 W. Michigan Street Indianapolis, IN 46202-3233 Phone: 317-637-9200	www.acsm.org	*Medicine & Science in Sports & Exercise Exercise and Sport Sciences Reviews Health & Fitness Journal*	Yes	$10
Academy of Nutrition and Dietetics	120 S. Riverside Plaza, Suite 2000 Chicago, IL 60606-6995 Phone: 800-877-1600	www.eatright.org	*Journal of the Academy of Nutrition and Dietetics Food and Nutrition Magazine Student Scoop Eat Right Weekly*	Yes	$50
American Institute of Wine and Food (AIWF)	26364 Carmel Rancho Lane, Suite 200E Carmel, CA 93923 Phone: 800-274-2493	www.aiwf.org	*American Food and Wine AIWF Newsletter*	No	Regular membership $75
American Public Health Association (APHA)	800 I Street, NW Washington, DC 20001 Phone: 202-777-274	www.apha.org	*American Journal of Public Health The Nation's Health*	Yes	$61
American Society for Nutrition	9650 Rockville Pike Bethesda, MD 20814-3998 Phone: 301-634-7050	www.nutrition.org	*The American Journal of Clinical Nutrition The Journal of Nutrition*	Yes	$30

(continues)

TABLE 8–2

Selected Professional Associations (Continued)

Organization	Address and Phone	Website Address	Publication(s) Available	Student Membership	Membership Dues
American Society for Parenteral and Enteral Nutrition (ASPEN)	8630 Fenton Street, Suite 412, Silver Spring, MD 20910, Phone: 301-587-2365	www.nutritioncare.org	*Journal of Parenteral and Enteral Nutrition*; *Nutrition in Clinical Practice*	Yes	$45
Association for Healthcare Foodservice (AHF)	455 S. 4th Street, Suite 650, Louisville, KY 40202, Phone: 888-528-9552	www.healthcarefoodservice.org	*Making an Informed Decision*; *S.O. Connected*	Yes	$25
Association of Nutrition and Foodservice Professionals	406 Surrey Woods Drive, St. Charles, IL 60174, Phone: 800-323-1908	www.anfponline.org	*Nutrition and Foodservice Edge*	Yes	$60
School Nutrition Association	120 Waterfront Street, Suite 300, National Harbor, MD 20745, Phone: 301-686-3100	www.asfsa.org	*School Nutrition Magazine.*; *Journal of Child Nutrition & Management*	Yes	$28
Society for Nutrition Education and Behavior (SNEB)	9100 Purdue Road, Suite 200, Indianapolis, IN 46268, Phone: 800-235-6690	www.sneb.org	*Journal of Nutrition Education & Behavior*; *The SNEB eCommunicator*	Yes	$60

Summary

Membership in the Academy of Nutrition and Dietetics, your state and district dietetic associations, Academy DPGs, or other professional associations or societies can enhance and enrich your professional and personal growth. Communication, networking, leadership opportunities, and other member benefits are available to those who participate. You determine your own level of involvement, and thus your own level of satisfaction. Become actively involved and reap the rewards of an active and involved professional life.

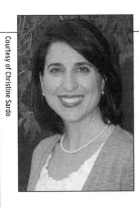

Courtesy of Christine Sardo

Profile of a Professional

Christine L. Sardo, MPH, RD

Partnerships and Policies Director
Canyon Ranch Institute
Tucson, Arizona

Education:
BS in Pre-Medicine and Nutrition, The Ohio State University, Columbus, Ohio
MPH, University of Minnesota, Minneapolis & St. Paul, Minnesota
National Institutes of Health Fellowship in Patient-Based Clinical Research—The Ohio State University, Columbus, Ohio

How did you first hear about dietetics and decide to become a Registered Dietitian?
I was first introduced to dietetics when I was a pre-med student and nutrition major at The Ohio State University. I was again introduced to the dietetics program while pursuing a master's in public health (MPH) degree in nutrition at the University of Minnesota.

What was your route to registration?
After almost a decade of working as a full-time professional, I decided to pursue my RD credential and was accepted into the dietetics internship at the Mount Carmel College of Nursing in Columbus, Ohio. I completed their 9-month internship program and successfully passed the registration exam shortly thereafter.

What are some examples of your professional involvement?
I am a member of the Academy of Nutrition and Dietetics and have been a speaker at the national Food & Nutrition Conference and Exhibition of the Academy. I've also been a board member of the Ohio Dietetic Association. In the local Columbus (OH) Dietetic Association, I served as public relations chairperson, president-elect, and president.

Have you received any awards or honors?
I was delighted to have been chosen as a Recognized Young Dietitian of the Year (RYDY) by the Ohio Dietetic Association.

Briefly describe your career path in dietetics. What are you doing now?
I currently lead partnership and policy functions for Canyon Ranch Institute (CRI), and I am the program manager for the Institute's partnerships with the Lance Armstrong Foundation and the Cleveland Clinic. CRI is a 501(c)(3) nonprofit organization. Our organization catalyzes the possibility of optimal health for all people by translating the best practices of CRI and its partners to help educate, inspire, and empower every person to prevent disease and choose a life of wellness.

Prior to joining CRI in February 2009, I managed the Cancer Chemoprevention Clinical Trials with black raspberries at The Ohio State University Comprehensive Cancer Center in Columbus, Ohio. I also served as a research and planning analyst for the Leo Burnett Company in Chicago and was a senior pharmaceutical representative for SmithKline Beecham and Janssen Pharmaceutica (Johnson & Johnson) in Columbus, Ohio. I also worked as a research assistant at the National Institutes of Health's National Heart, Lung and Blood Institute. Collaborating with the public and professional colleagues, I have developed educational seminars, articles, videos, and cooking demonstrations to improve health literacy about how we can all achieve optimal wellness. For example, in addition to my leadership role at CRI, I also serve as the nutrition and cancer prevention and survivorship expert for LIVESTRONG.com. I regularly contribute articles, post blogs, and answer readers' questions about how to prevent cancer through nutrition.

In addition, I have taught cancer prevention and survivorship seminars and have led educational sessions in the United States and internationally. Among those presentations, I am particularly pleased to have had the opportunity to present at The Ohio State University Lance Armstrong Center of Excellence; Dr. Andrew Weil's Nutrition and Health: State of the Science and Clinical Applications conference; Canyon Ranch; the Academy of Nutrition and Dietetics's National Food and Nutrition Conference and Exhibition; and Peking University Health Sciences Center in Beijing, China. I have authored and coauthored several nutrition and chemoprevention articles for the public and for peer-reviewed publications, including the *Journal of Clinical Pharmacology, Seminars in Cancer Biology*, and *Cancer Epidemiology Biomarkers and Prevention*. I was also a contributor to the *National Call to Action on Cancer Prevention and Survivorship*.

What excites you about dietetics and the future of our profession?
With mounting evidence showing the link between nutrition and cancer, as well as other conditions, translating the science into meaningful messages that resonate with the public is an exciting area for the future of our profession. Also, it will be very interesting and exciting to see the emerging field of nutrigenomics unfold, as research that further elucidates the relationship between food, our genes, and risk for disease continues to evolve.

What words of wisdom do you have for future dietetics professionals?
Stay positive and make the best of every opportunity. Always stay abreast of the newest research and findings in nutrition and health. Finally, always stay connected with your peers and colleagues.

Suggested Activities

1. Attend a district, state, or national dietetics meeting and share your impressions with your instructor and classmates.

2. Look for the issue of the *Journal of the Academy of Nutrition and Dietetics* that showcases the new officers of the Academy. Read the brief description about each person and find out in what area of dietetics each person works.

3. Are you a student member of the Academy of Nutrition and Dietetics? If so, have you visited the members-only Student Center online at www.eatright.org? What kind of information is found there? If you are not a member, consider joining.

4. Who are the officers of your state dietetic association? What kinds of dietetics positions do they hold? How often does the state association meet?

5. Invite your state's delegate(s) from the Academy's House of Delegates to your class to talk about current issues relevant to dietetics.

6. Which DPGs or MIGs in the Academy of Nutrition and Dietetics are of most interest to you? Visit the website of your top three and look at the membership benefits of each group. How much does it cost to become a member of each group?

7. Does your school have a student nutrition and dietetics club? If so, do you actively participate? If not, attend the next meeting and find out what is going on. If your school does not have a student nutrition and dietetics club, get together with your classmates and form one. Contact other schools that have dietetics programs to find out if they have a nutrition and dietetics club and what types of activities they sponsor.

Selected Websites

- www.eatright.org—The Academy of Nutrition and Dietetics, the world's largest organization of food and nutrition professionals
- www.cnmdpg.org—Clinical Nutrition Management Dietetic Practice Group
- www.dce.org—Diabetes Care and Education Dietetic Practice Group
- www.depdpg.org—Nutrition and Dietetic Educators and Preceptors Dietetic Practice Group
- www.dtpdpg.org—Dietetic Technicians in Practice Dietetic Practice Group
- www.dnsdpg.org—Dietitians in Nutrition Support Dietetic Practice Group
- www.foodculinaryprofs.org—Food and Culinary Professionals Dietetic Practice Group
- www.hendpg.com—Hunger and Environmental Nutrition Dietetic Practice Group
- www.nepdpg.org—Nutrition Education for the Public Dietetic Practice Group
- www.nehpdpg.org—Nutrition Educators of Health Professionals Dietetic Practice Group
- www.nedpg.org—Nutrition Entrepreneurs Dietetic Practice Group
- www.oncologynutrition.org—Oncology Nutrition Dietetic Practice Group
- www.pnpg.org—Pediatric Nutrition Dietetic Practice Group
- www.renalnutrition.org—Renal Dietitians Dietetic Practice Group
- www.scandpg.org—Sports, Cardiovascular, and Wellness Nutrition Dietetic Practice Group
- http://vegetariannutrition.net—Vegetarian Nutrition Dietetic Practice Group

- http://wmdpg.org—Weight Management Dietetic Practice Group
- http://womenshealthdpg.org—Women's Health Dietetic Practice Group

References

1. American Dietetic Association. *Promoting Better Health Through Better Nutrition.* Chicago: The American Dietetic Association, 1995.

2. Cassell JA. *Carry the Flame: The History of the American Dietetic Association.* Chicago: The American Dietetic Association, 1990.

3. American Dietetic Association. Membership Classification Information. Available at: http://www.eatright.org. Accessed October 23, 2009.

4. American Dietetic Association. Honorary Membership. Available at: http://www.eatright.org. Accessed October 23, 2009.

5. American Dietetic Association. What is ADA? Available at: http://www.eatright.org. Accessed October 23, 2009.

6. American Dietetic Association. ADA Foundation. Available at: http://www.eatright.org. Accessed October 23, 2009.

7. American Dietetic Association. Commission on Dietetic Registration. Available at: http://www.eatright.org. Accessed October 23, 2009.

8. American Dietetic Association. Government Affairs. Available at: http://www.eatright.org. Accessed October 23, 2009.

9. American Dietetic Association. Board of Directors. Available at: http://www.eatright.org. Accessed October 23, 2009.

10. American Dietetic Association. House of Delegates. Available at: http://www.eatright.org. Accessed October 23, 2009.

11. American Dietetic Association. Affiliates. Available at: http://www.eatright.org. Accessed October 23, 2009.

12. American Dietetic Association. Dietetic Practice Groups. Available at: http://www.eatright.org. Accessed October 23, 2009.

13. American Dietetic Association. Marjorie Hulsizer Copher Award. Available at: http://www.eatright.org. Accessed October 23, 2009.

14. American Dietetic Association. Lenna Frances Cooper Lecturer. Available at: http://www.eatright.org. Accessed October 23, 2009.

15. American Dietetic Association. Medallion Award. Available at: http://www.eatright.org. Accessed October 23, 2009.

16. American Dietetic Association. ADAF Awards for Excellence in Practice. Available at: http://www.eatright.org. Accessed October 23, 2009.

17. American Dietetic Association. Member Benefits. Available at: http://www.eatright.org. Accessed October 23, 2009.

18. Academy of Nutrition and Dietetics. Current Overview. Available at http://www.eatright.org. Accessed April 30, 2012.

The Future

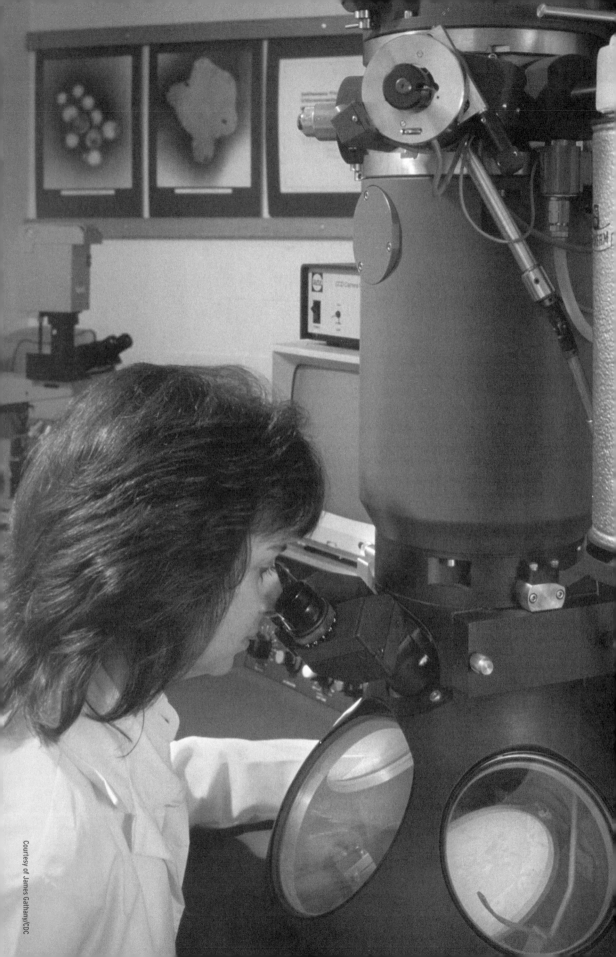

Trends, Predictions, and Your Future

If we had a crystal ball and could look into the future, what would we see for the future of dietetics? What roles will dietitians play? What areas of practice that are unheard of now, will exist in the years ahead? What will be the impact of technology on the practice of dietetics? Will the future needs of our clients be different from what they are today?

In 2010, the Workforce Demand Task Force of what was then the American Dietetic Association identified 10 change drivers that they predicted would influence the future of the dietetics workforce and demand for dietetics services. The results of this "Future Scan" were published in a special supplement of the March 2012 issue of the *Journal of the Academy of Nutrition and Dietetics*.[1] The results of this study are most revealing.

The change drivers identified by the Task Force are:

- An aging population will create both challenges and opportunities for dietetics professionals.
- Growing diversity in the U.S. population will bring new challenges to a very nondiverse population of dietetics practitioners who may lack the necessary cross-cultural skills and knowledge to serve them.
- A growing and more diverse student population interested in dietetics will expect dietetics education to provide them with immediate and sustainable employment.
- Dietitians must become a critical part of the growing trend toward interdisciplinary teams in the arenas where nutrition is important. Knowing how to work as a team and solve problems will be more important than competencies and credentials.
- Employers will value adaptable generalists more than specialists. Dietetics practitioners must be ready to take advantage of emerging opportunities rather than specializing in areas that may be declining in importance.

- Technology will become increasingly important in client interaction and counseling and dietetics practitioners must be on the cutting-edge.
- Personalized nutrition will require even higher levels of scientific knowledge and technical skill as new opportunities evolve for dietetics professionals.
- The healthfulness, safety, and sustainability of the food supply chain are ongoing concerns of the food industry and the public. A steady supply of dietetics professionals who are trained to work in this arena is lacking and this need must be addressed.
- While the future of healthcare reform is still uncertain, dietetics professionals must be ready to prove their value in both health promotion and disease prevention.

Because of the increase in chronic disease, obesity, and socioeconomic challenges, more dietetic professionals are needed to work in new practice roles associated with nutrition initiatives and life-course interventions.[1]

The Change Drivers and Their Implications for Dietetics Practice

Although trends are interesting to explore, this doesn't mean they will necessarily materialize. No one has yet discovered how to predict the future! However, the systematic forecast of trends and patterns by futurists is critical to planning—whether for a professional organization or for one's personal future. Following is a synopsis of predicted societal changes and their possible effects on dietetics practice.

Change Driver #1: The Aging of America

The fact that the average age of the U.S. population is steadily increasing is no surprise. The 2010 U.S. Census predicted that between 2000 and 2020, the elderly population in our country will grow by over 36%. Because of this trend, the dietetics profession has a huge role to play in helping these individuals maintain or improve their nutritional status and overall quality of life. This changing demographic is also going to impact the profession itself. Some older dietetics professionals will make the decision to retire, which may leave critical shortages in some areas of dietetics practice. On the other hand, other older professionals may decide to keep working past what we consider the typical retirement age.

The dietetics profession is expected to experience an attrition rate of 2–5%. This rate coupled with the estimated growth of the over-65 population by 120% by 2050, means growing job opportunities in gerontology but a decreasing supply of dietetics practitioners.[2] Because older people are at a higher risk for chronic diseases such as cancer, diabetes, cardiovascular diseases, and osteoporosis, the need for dietetics services is only going to grow as the elderly population soars with the retirement of the Baby Boomer generation.

Workforce opportunities for dietetics professionals include:

- "Increased demand for geriatric care, especially in institutional settings.
- Older career changers may consider nutrition careers.
- Businesses offering wellness programs for senior workers."[1]

Change Driver #2: Population and Workforce Diversity

Immigration in the U.S. has increased significantly in the last 20 years, resulting in many new immigrant communities across our country. For the first time, racial and ethnic minorities now make up more than half of the children born in the United States causing a shift in our country's racial makeup.[3] Such a shift speaks to the increasing need for cultural competence among dietetics professionals and to recruit new dietetics professionals from among these racial and ethnic groups. Many of these growing ethnic communities exhibit poor health related to diet, exercise, and socioeconomic factors. Programs targeting behavior change in schools and other community venues will be critical.[1]

Currently, an estimated 84% of RDs and 81% of DTRs are non-Hispanic white and 96% of RDs and 95% of DTRs are women.[2] This diversity gap must be addressed if the dietetics profession is going to successfully serve an ever-increasing diverse population.

Workforce opportunities for dietetics professionals include:

- "Poor nutrition will drive demand for community dietetics practitioners.
- Foodservice and consulting dietetics practitioners will be vital to improving school food programs.
- Increased funding for chronic disease prevention will drive demand for dietetics practitioners."[1]

Change Driver #3: Workforce Education

Job changes are common in a person's working career, and often individuals who have been in a particular career for many years look for new opportunities.[4] Because of the growing interest in nutrition and health, more and more individuals are interested in dietetics as a second career. Healthcare jobs are considered a growth area in what has been a sluggish economy.[5] Online education makes pursuing continuing education or new career education even more convenient. A growing number of online dietetic education programs and "distance internships" may help make dietetics an even more attractive alternative for those seeking a new career.

Currently the career path into dietetics is a very prescribed process and competition, particularly for the supervised practice component, is fierce. If the supply of dietetics professionals is going to meet the predicted need, dietetics education must become even more flexible, with a more seamless transition between education and supervised practice, if the profession is going to attract the new entrants it needs.

Workforce opportunities for dietetics professionals include:

- "Interprofessional learning could expand the number of dietetics and nutrition specialists.
- Healthcare career opportunities are growing and are perceived as more secure."[1]

Change Driver #4: Interdisciplinary Teaming Drives Innovation

Dietetics professionals must learn to work even more collaboratively with other healthcare team members. Whether working on research problems, developing new products, or enhancing patient care, interdisciplinary teams are increasingly important in today's healthcare environment. Dietetics professionals must be ready to step up and assume leadership on these interdisciplinary teams, whether working in clinical nutrition, in health promotion/disease prevention, or in foodservice systems management.[1]

If dietetics practitioners are going to be comfortable working with various healthcare team members in patient-centered care teams, interdisciplinary training must begin during dietetics education. ACEND core knowledge and competencies stress the importance of dietetics students/interns sharing learning experiences with other health professions students during their education and training.

Workforce opportunities for dietetics professionals include:

- "Nutrition is central to health and critical to solving many health-related challenges.
- Registered dietitians can assume new roles as team leaders and coordinators.
- Teaming could bring together the three primary sectors of dietetics: clinical, health promotion/disease prevention, and food production and foodservice."[1]

Change Driver #5: Generalists Gain an Edge on Specialists

According to the Future Scan report, "New entrants to the dietetics profession will need to be broadly educated for careers that will morph many times to meet new demands for food and nutrition expertise."[1] The Academy's core knowledge and competencies form a strong basis for entry into dietetics. The future calls for dietetics practitioners who will build on this foundation and diversify their career portfolios with a variety of experiences where leadership skills and project knowledge are honed.

The issues of specialty practice and advanced practice in dietetics are "hot topics." Does the pursuit of specialty credentials fly in the face of this prediction that generalists with an interdisciplinary perspective and leadership skills are more highly valued by employers? How is an "advanced practitioner" different from a specialist? What are the continuing education needs of specialty and advanced dietetics practitioners and how can this continuing education best be provided? All of these are important questions that must be addressed in the days ahead.

Workforce opportunities for dietetics professionals include:

- "RDs can migrate with health care out of the clinical setting.
- RDs may be a step ahead in adopting the skills to lead interdisciplinary teams.
- Management opportunities offer better compensation and career growth."[1]

Change Driver #6: Technology Transforms Nutrition Counseling

Advances in technology have totally transformed how we live, how we learn, and how we communicate. Because of the avalanche of information, that is available to consumers from a single Google search, patients or clients may come to a nutrition counseling session armed with an abundance of information, which may or may not be accurate. The dietetics professional must be the translator or interpreter who helps their patient or client make sense of it all.

The ways in which technology may be used to communicate nutrition information and stay in touch with customers, clients, and/or patients is limited only by one's imagination. The use of social media and other technological communication tools will enable healthcare providers and their patients to interact and stay in touch no matter where they are in the world. Never before have we had such capability to collect, monitor, and interpret health data at a moment's notice. Whether using the Internet, iPads, smart phones or other yet-undreamed-of technologies, the capabilities for nutrition and lifestyle intervention and counseling seem virtually limitless. Dietetics professionals need to be continually updating themselves on such new technologies as well as helping to create them.

Workforce opportunities for dietetics professionals include:

- "Demand for nutrition information in food systems will increase.
- Expert systems can improve patient care and free time for dietitians to provide higher-value services.
- Virtual worlds will provide more avenues to reach and influence patients.
- Advanced modeling and simulation technology will allow greater personalization of diet plans."[1]

Change Driver #7: Personalized Nutrition Evolves

It appears that finally we are seeing a shift in the focus of our healthcare system from one that treats disease to a system that focuses on prediction and prevention. The human genome project has led to the field of nutritional genomics or nutrigenomics. According to the Center of Excellence for Nutritional Genomics at the University of California, Davis, **nutrigenomics** is "the study of how foods affect our genes and how individual genetic differences can affect the way we respond to nutrients in the foods we eat."[6] Nutrition counseling is an important part of nutrigenomics and the shift to health promotion/disease prevention, leading to new opportunities for dietetics professionals.

Technology has also provided the way for patients and their healthcare providers to monitor an individual's health at home or away from home. Data collected in this way for whole communities will provide an important scientific base for studying the outcomes of dietary or other interventions. Dietitians should be actively involved in this kind of ongoing research.

Screening for genetic disorders is becoming more and more common, and this will create new opportunities for advanced practice RDs who are trained in genetics. Early intervention and counseling can prevent serious or even life-threatening disabilities.

Workforce opportunities for dietetics professionals include:

- Early testing will identify the best candidates for nutrition intervention and counseling, thereby expanding reimbursement for these services.

- Better outcomes research will shift funds to prevention rather than treatment, creating more demand for nutrition counseling and intervention.
- Opportunities for dietetics practitioners will appear first in sports nutrition and geriatric care."[1]

Change Driver #8: Food Industry Transforms for Public Priorities

Today's consumers are becoming more interested in healthful eating, where their food is coming from, and how it has been handled during its production. The companies that make up the food industry recognize that they must be ready to answer consumer questions, respond to consumer preferences, and meet the government's demands for industry support of public health. As the Workforce Demand Task Force report indicates, while "price, convenience, and marketing still make or break food businesses, consumers are less willing to give up these advantages at the expense of health, safety, and sustainability."[1]

There are exciting opportunities in the future for dietetics professionals to work in the food industry in roles such as public relations, marketing, research and development, sales, or directing nutrition communications for food companies. A new requirement in the healthcare reform law mandates that restaurants provide nutrition information on their menus, and dietetics professionals are uniquely qualified to help restaurants with this challenge.

Workforce opportunities for dietetics professionals include:

- "Entrepreneurial niches will open up for risk-takers."
- "These career opportunities might make the dietetics profession attractive to people with business and environmental interests."
- "Food is a necessity and jobs will always exist for those who provide it."[1]

Change Drivers #9 and #10: Healthcare Reform Boosts Access to Dietetics Services; Uncertainty of Public Support and Funding for Health Initiatives and Prevention Strategies

The final two change drivers identified by the Workforce Demand Task Force are challenging to discuss. At the time of this writing, President Obama's healthcare reform legislation is being challenged in the U.S. Supreme Court. The outcome of the Court's deliberation is unknown. Because the healthcare reform law focuses more on health promotion/disease prevention, its implementation could provide dietetics professionals the opportunity to be vitally important players in the new healthcare paradigm. However, the legislation does not ensure that dietetics practitioners will be the only healthcare team members providing nutrition services.

Public support and funding for health initiatives and prevention strategies is very uncertain. Because our society suffers from widespread chronic disease, obesity, and other challenges, nutrition interventions led by dietetics professionals must be a priority for the future health of our nation. Only time will tell if public support and sufficient dietetics practitioners will be available to meet the challenge.[1]

The Future for Dietetics Professionals

According to the Bureau of Labor Statistics of the U.S. Department of Labor, the job market for dietetics professionals continues to grow, with a projected growth rate of 20% from 2010–2020, faster than the average for all occupations.[7] According to the Department of Labor, job growth will result from an increasing emphasis on disease prevention through improved dietary habits. A growing and aging population will boost demand for nutritional counseling and treatment in hospitals, residential care facilities, schools, prisons, community health programs, and home healthcare agencies. Public interest in nutrition and increased emphasis on health education and prudent lifestyles will also spur demand, especially in foodservice management. Entrepreneurs such as personal chefs and trainers who prepare and cook food for clients in their homes and give personal nutrition advice are challenging dietetics professionals. Some dietitians are seeking additional credentials, such as those discussed in Chapter 7, to broaden the services they are able to deliver. Dietitians are also gaining new knowledge and skills in disciplines such as pharmacy, exercise physiology, biochemistry, culinary arts, communication, business, and other areas.

The Final Report of the Phase 2 Future Dietetics Practice and Education Task Force in 2008 spelled out a description of the future DTR, the future entry-level RD, and the future advanced-practice RD in a variety of practice areas.[8]

The Future Dietetic Technician, Registered

According to the task force report, the DTR is an important and vital member of the dietetics team. That team may include foodservice workers, Certified Dietary Managers (CDMs), RDs, RD specialists, and advanced-practice RDs. DTRs are predicted to function in specialty areas with the RD. The DTR will work in the delivery of food and nutrition services in a wide variety of settings, including such activities as supervising food production and service systems, providing community outreach, conducting nutrition education and food demonstrations, working on meal analysis and recipe development, conducting diet histories for clinical care and research, participating in continuous quality improvement, and using technology to enhance practice. Using the Nutrition Care Process, the DTR will be actively engaged in health promotion and disease prevention through identification of specific client or community needs. DTRs practice as directed by or under the supervision of the RD in the nutrition care process and may function with a varying degree of autonomy depending on the complexity of foodservice operations.[8]

The Future Entry-Level RD

The task force identified roles for the entry-level RD in a wide range of practice areas including generalist, health promotion/disease prevention, public policy, clinical health care, education, research, food production and service management, and the food industry. A common theme among all of these roles is that the entry-level RD as an important and contributing member of a team. No matter what role the entry-level RD fills, certain foundational practice elements must also be present:

- Provision of patient/client-centered care.
- Use of evidence-based recommendations and professional judgment to challenge the status quo.
- Contribution is made to the body of knowledge by participating in operational analyses, business process improvement, and other applied research activities and by monitoring and evaluating the effectiveness of the nutrition care provided and reporting results.
- Analysis, interpretation, and application of research.
- Adoption of technology advancements.
- Utilization of informatics.
- Demonstration of leadership in multidisciplinary teams.
- Contribution to the advancement of food and nutrition policy through advocacy.[8]

The Future Advanced-Level RD

The knowledge and skills outlined for an advanced-practice RD comprise a common core, including nutrition and food sciences, leadership, food composition and preparation, management principles and concepts, communication and information technology, business practice management, marketing, research methodologies and statistics, regulatory compliance, grant writing, food safety, scientific inquiry, human resources development and management, finance and budgeting, and organizational development and administration.

Practice settings for advanced-practice RDs include clinical health care, higher education, health promotion/disease prevention, food and/or food production and service systems, public policy, and research.[8]

Summary

The future of dietetics is dynamic and exciting. Entrepreneurial dietitians, who see change as opportunity, will be the ones who take dietetics through the next century. Dietitians must be willing to seize opportunities to market themselves and their abilities in new and exciting ways. If we are to fulfill the Academy's vision to optimize the nation's health through food and nutrition and the Academy's mission to empower members to be the nation's food and nutrition leaders,[9] we must look to the future with energy, enthusiasm, and an entrepreneurial spirit. The profession of dietetics has a bright and exciting future. Only your energy level and imagination will limit you. Prepare now to be a part of that bright future!

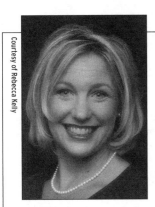

Profile of a Professional

Rebecca K. Kelly, PhD, RD, CDE

Assistant Professor and Director
Office of Health Promotion and Wellness
The University of Alabama
Tuscaloosa, Alabama
President, Element Health, Inc.
Birmingham, Alabama

Education:
BS in Nutrition and Food Science, Auburn University, Auburn,
    Alabama
MA in Education with an emphasis in Exercise Physiology, The
    University of Alabama, Tuscaloosa, Alabama
PhD in Health Education and Health Promotion, The University of Alabama,
    Birmingham, Alabama
Dietetic internship—Indiana University Medical Center, Indianapolis, Indiana

How did you first hear about dietetics and decide to become a Registered Dietitian?
As a college student–athlete, I was drawn to the profession of nutrition at it relates to
performance in athletics and adults.

What are some examples of your professional involvement?
Professional involvement has been through the Academy of Nutrition and Dietetics,
in Dietetic Practice Groups, and in my local dietetic association. I've been a member
of both the Birmingham and Tuscaloosa District Dietetic Associations, and served as
public relations chair for the Birmingham organization. I'm also active in other groups
that complement my dietetics interest, including the Alabama Conference on Obesity,
the Health Enhancement Research Organization Think Tank, the Wellness Councils
of America national panel of advisors, the State of Alabama Diabetes Network as an
executive committee member, the Alabama Lung Association, the Governor's Task
Force on Physical Activity, and the American Sports Medicine Institute Sports and
Science Camp steering committee.

What honors and awards have you received?
I've been the recipient of numerous scholarships during my academic journey, includ-
ing scholarships from the Academy of Nutrition and Dietetics and the Alabama
Dietetic Association. I was honored as The University of Alabama at Birmingham School
of Education Alumnus of the Year, The University of Alabama at Birmingham, Depart-
ment of Health Education and Physical Education Outstanding Graduate Student,
Auburn University's Centennial of Women Outstanding Woman Graduate, and Auburn
University President's Award recipient.

Briefly describe your career path in dietetics. What are you doing now?
After completing both my undergraduate degree and dietetic internship, I spent
approximately 2 years practicing as a Registered Dietitian in clinical settings
in Indianapolis and Birmingham. I then returned to graduate school at The
University of Alabama, where I served as a graduate research assistant in the
field of exercise physiology. Upon graduating with my master's degree, I began
the consulting firm Element Health, Inc., previously NEWtrition Connection, a specialty nutrition and wellness consulting company based in Birmingham, Alabama.
Today, this company employs a network of healthcare professionals, including

registered dietitians, and serves individuals as well as corporate and government clients with the provision of high-quality clinical nutrition, wellness, and sports nutrition services.

Following the launch of my consulting business, I worked for 13 years as the wellness manager at American Cast Iron Pipe Company, named by *Fortune* magazine as one of the top 100 best companies to work for in America. In 2007, I seized an opportunity for growth and am now putting my nutrition, exercise, diabetes, and management knowledge and experience to work for the benefit of employees at The University of Alabama, serving as the director of Health Promotion and Wellness.

What excites you about dietetics and the future of our profession?
The growing opportunities available to those in the field of nutrition and dietetics excite me most. The growing population—in age and number—creates a greater opportunity for dietitians in all settings. I wish to encourage all dietitians to be open to the many new and expanding opportunities and roles that are ever-changing and creatively available.

Why/how is teamwork important to you in your position? How have you been involved in team projects?
People working together in groups can do much more than individuals alone; good teamwork is vital to furthering the agenda of any strategic program for improving health and wellness. I have participated in a variety of teams with many different agendas, and, although I am effective in a supportive role, I find my true strength and interests lie in leadership positions. My joy lies in envisioning and designing new strategies and programs to push the team forward toward achieving positive outcomes.

What words of wisdom do you have for future dietetics professionals?
Find your passion! Be open to opportunities to connect your interests, knowledge, and skills to more fully develop and define our profession, while making a difference in the health and lives of others.

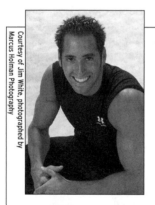

Profile of a Professional

Jim White, RD, ACSM-HFS

Owner
Jim White Fitness and Nutrition Studios
Virginia Beach, Virginia

Education:
BS in Dietetics, Youngstown State University, Youngstown, Ohio
Coordinated Program in Dietetics

Where did you first learn about dietetics and decide to become a Registered Dietitian?
My first exposure to dietetics was from talking to a college professor.

What was your route to registration?
I graduated *summa cum laude* from the Coordinated Program in Dietetics at Youngstown State University in Youngstown, Ohio. My bachelor of science in applied science degree combined the required dietetics coursework with the supervised practice experience, which I did at Northside Hospital in Youngstown.

What has been your career path in dietetics, and what are you doing now?

After college, I became credentialed as a Registered Dietitian and certified by the American College of Sports Medicine as an exercise specialist. I moved to Virginia Beach where I started my own personal training business, JDW Fitness and Nutrition, LLC. I gained additional exposure when I began competing in body-building competitions and running marathons across the country and by holding nutrition and fitness seminars. Some of my other projects include a fitness reality show, a fitness video, a health-related magazine, and my own line of supplements and fitness apparel. I recently self-published my first book entitled, *The JW Fit-in-30 Plan*. I've been fortunate to have opportunities to be nationally featured on the ABC Family Channel's *The 700 Club* and *Living the Life, TLC, Radio Disney*, and the Discovery Channel. I've also written articles on nutrition and fitness for *Men's Health, Men's Fitness, Oxygen, Maximum Fitness, Better Homes and Gardens*, Newsweek.com, Forbes.com, USNews.com, CNN.com, *New Body*, and *Wine Spectator*.

On November 1, 2005, I opened Jim White Fitness Studios on Shore Drive in Virginia Beach, Virginia, and have opened up two more studios, one in 2006 and another in 2009. My future plans are to open a chain of branded Jim White Fitness Studios nationwide.

Are you involved in professional organizations?

I am currently a spokesperson for the Academy of Nutrition and Dietetics, speaking on men's health, weight loss, fad diets, and sports nutrition. I'm also a regional spokesman for the Alzheimer's Association and have teamed up with the national Junior League as their chairman to tackle the childhood obesity epidemic. I've been president of the Tidewater Dietetic Association and have served on the board of directors for the Virginia Dietetic Association. I was fortunate to have been selected as the Recognized Young Dietitian of the Year (RYDY) for Virginia in 2009.

What excites you about dietetics and the future of our profession?

The possibilities are endless! So many people need to develop better eating habits to improve their walk in life!

What words of wisdom do you have for future dietetics professionals?

Nothing is impossible. There will be many who are against you, but stick to your values and dreams, and move forward. There will be many supporting you. Take their advice and use it to fuel you. Above all, believe in yourself and never give up!

Suggested Activities

1. Review copies of the *Journal of the Academy of Nutrition and Dietetics* and the Academy's *Food & Nutrition* magazine for the past year. What hot topics are being discussed in these publications? How much do you know about these topics? How do you think these topics may affect your future practice in dietetics?

2. Read current issues of popular newspapers or newsmagazines, such as *The Wall Street Journal, Time, Newsweek,* and so on. Look specifically for articles that might relate to dietetic practice, including topics related to health, food, nutrition, foodservice, public health, and others. What implications might these topics have for dietetics?

3. Review the "President's Page" in each issue of the *Journal of the Academy of Nutrition and Dietetics.* What topics have been discussed? What issues are facing the profession of dietetics or the Academy of Nutrition and Dietetics?

4. Search online for the websites of some entrepreneurial dietitians and see what kinds of services they provide. Some websites of entrepreneurial dietitians are provided in the following "Selected Websites" section.

Selected Websites

- www.nancyclarkrd.com—Nancy Clark, MS, RD, CSSD, is an internationally known sports nutritionist and best-selling author trusted by many top athletes.
- www.nutritionexpert.com—Mitzi Dulan, RD, CSSD, is a nutrition and health spokesperson, author, and speaker.
- http://xn--www-rp0a.healthykidschallenge.com/—HKC is a nationally recognized 501(c)3 nonprofit led by registered licensed dietitians with years of school, program, and community wellness experience.
- www.susanmitchell.org—Susan Mitchell, PhD, RD, FADA, is a nutrition spokesperson, consultant, and author/freelance writer.
- www.ellynsatter.com/—Ellyn Satter, MS, RD, LCSW, BCD, at Ellyn Satter Associates provides resources for professionals and the public in the area of eating and feeding.
- http://nutritionforkids.com/24_Carrot.htm—24 Carrot Press publishes titles that promote the nutritional health of children and adolescents.

References

1. Rhea M, Bettles C. Future changes driving dietetics workforce supply and demand: Future scan 2012–2022. *J Acad Nutr and Dietetics* 2012;S10–S24.

2. Compensation and Benefits Survey of the Dietetics Profession 2011. Chicago, IL: American Dietetic Association.

3. Yen H. Minority birth rate now surpasses whites in U.S., census shows. Available at http://www.huffingtonpost.com/2012/05/17/minorities-birth-rate-now-surpass-whites-in-us-census_n_1523230.html. Accessed May 20, 2012.

4. Bialik C. Seven careers in a lifetime? Think twice, researchers say. Available at http://online.wsj.com/article/SB10001424052748704206804575468162805877990.html. Accessed May 20, 2012.

5. Kavilanz P. Health care jobs a bright spot for hiring. Available at http://money.cnn.com/2011/07/08/news/economy/healthcare_jobs/index.htm. Accessed May 20, 2012.

6. The NCMHD Center of Excellence for Nutritional Genomics, University of California, Davis. Available at http://nutrigenomics.ucdavis.edu/?page=Information. Accessed May 23, 2012.

7. U.S. Department of Labor, Bureau of Labor Statistics. *Occupational Outlook Handbook*, 2010–2011. Dietitians and nutritionists. Available at: http://www.bls.gov/oco/ocos077 .htm#emply. Accessed May 23, 2012.

8. American Dietetic Association. Final Report of the Phase 2 Future Dietetics Practice and Education Task Force, July 15, 2008. Available at: http://www.eatright.org/Members /content.aspx?id=8347. Accessed May 23, 2012.

9. The Academy's Strategic Plan: Mission and Vision. Available at: http://www.eatright.org /strategicplan/. Accessed May 23, 2012.

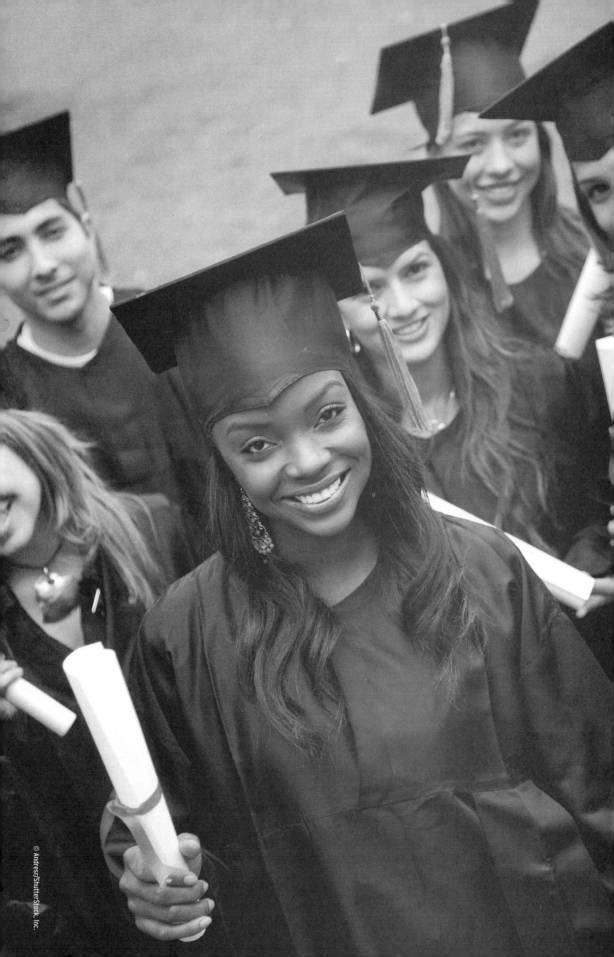

Crossing the Bridge: From Student to Professional

Are you ready for the real world? When you arrived on campus as a freshman, your goal may have been survival—academic and social. With the voluminous amount of reading and writing required by your classes, seemingly endless time spent in labs, juggling the demands of work and school, and fitting in some extracurricular activities, very little time is left to think about the next step. Until senior year, when reality hits! What's next—graduate school, work, internship, marriage, family, travel, money? Where, when, and how decisions. This can be a very stressful time, not only because of the important decisions that must be made, but also because of the changes that must be faced. What will be the same and what will be different when you leave college to enter your profession? How difficult will it be to cross that bridge? And how can you make the transition successfully?

Transitions, in general, are challenging periods of one's life, whether it is elementary to middle school, high school to college, undergraduate to graduate school, graduate school to a professional life, reentering the professional world after taking time off, or changing career paths. This chapter focuses on the transition from school to profession, with the realization that it may be somewhat different in every case. For some, it may be more challenging than for others. For most, however, some strategies to manage the stresses associated with the changes that are faced can lay the foundation for career success. Engaging in self-assessment and developing clearly defined career goals, as discussed in Chapter 4, compose the first step.

How does the student role differ from the professional role? If you are reading this text, you are already familiar with the student role. So, what does it mean to be a professional? Consider someone whom you would describe as professional. If you were asked to describe this person, what would you say? Would you say that he or she is knowledgeable, ethical, caring, well dressed and well groomed, competent, assertive, responsible, committed to work and profession, a team player, and respectful of others? In this chapter, we examine the conduct, aims, and qualities considered characteristic of the dietetics profession. We emphasize the importance of showing respect and concern for people, being knowledgeable and keeping current with the latest research in one's area of practice, adhering to the strictest ethical standards, and having a commitment to the profession.

Professional Advice

The consistent piece of advice from those who have been there is that you need to figure out how to make the transition from student to professional while you are still in school, and the earlier the better. "Figuring it out" includes defining your career goals, making a commitment to manage your future, identifying a mentor, utilizing networking opportunities, and taking some risks.

Self-assessment and determining career goals are discussed in Chapter 4 "Beginning Your Path to Success in Dietetics." With some definite, possible, tentative, or interesting career goals in mind, the next step is to decide which internships, graduate programs, or companies and jobs can help you to achieve these goals. Research possibilities early in your college career to determine what knowledge, skills, work experience, and other qualities will make you a good candidate for your choices. This information will be helpful in making decisions on elective courses, fieldwork experiences, part-time jobs, extracurricular activities, service learning, and volunteer opportunities.

Seeking out professional advice should also occur early in your college career. The obvious way to seek professional advice is to talk to professionals. As a student, you have the opportunity to talk to professors in the field. Some students are reluctant to approach professors and instead wait for them to offer help. This is one time that it may be necessary to take the initiative. Professors are busy people, too, juggling departmental, professional, and personal demands on their time. But most faculty members want to help students in their program. You simply have to ask.

Interviewing dietetic practitioners who work in the areas of practice in which you are interested may also be helpful. In addition to taking the initiative to create some informal interactions with professors and other professionals, it is a good idea to take advantage of the student memberships offered by most professional associations. The printed materials that are sent to members can give you a good overview of the field, issues faced by the profession, current job listings, research being conducted, and calendars of professional events that provide networking and professional development opportunities.

Developing a relationship with a professional of a more formal nature, a mentor, can provide invaluable help during the transition as well as during the early stages of a career transition. A **mentor** is a wise and trusted counselor and guide. Mentoring is a special kind of caring, supportive relationship or partnership between two people based on trust and respect. Mentors share their knowledge and experience with mentees (protégés) to help them define and reach their goals. Faculty members and preceptors often serve as early mentors to students (**Figure 10–1**).

According to the late Pauline Schatz, EdD, RD, a longtime proponent of mentoring:

> *Positive relationships benefit the mentor, mentee, and society. In a nurturing relationship the mentor finds gratification providing guidance for the mentee to reach his/her goals. The mentee meets with a role model who motivates and guides the mentee toward the fulfillment of possibilities and personal goals. By practicing in a safe, stable environment, the mentee gains confidence while developing new skills. Both mentor and mentee are able to assess their knowledge and experience as well as take advantage of the opportunity for self-reflection. This results in a higher level of productivity. Society benefits not only from the increased productivity but also in this relationship the mentor, through the mentee, is often able to develop a legacy for future leadership that in turn will provide guidance for a new generation.*[1]

Although mentoring has been traditionally a one-on-one relationship, the team approach can be applied here as well. "Talent teams" have been formed to offer professional advice, to help solve problems, and to provide opportunities for collaboration or referrals, stimulation, and encouragement. A talent team is essentially organized lateral mentoring. Just like traditional mentoring, it involves a commitment to sharing time and information. The difference is that everyone is on the same level, and all ideas and feedback are of equal importance and consideration. Such a team may include a nutrition educator, a behavior change consultant, a national healthcare consultant, a communications consultant, a product development manager, and a marketing and research consultant.[2]

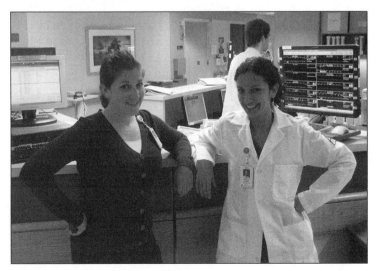

FIGURE 10–1 An intern and her clinical preceptor meet.
Courtesy of Michele Coelho, RD

You Are Entering a Helping Profession

By its very nature, dietetics is a helping profession. Dietetic practice involves service. The way this service is delivered is critically important. Respect, caring, and concern for people and their value systems are basic to the concept of professionalism. These characteristics may be manifested in many ways, not the least of which is respect for the dignity of each and every person. An understanding of individual differences, such as gender, ethnicity, and religion, is also critical for effective practice.

Lifelong Learning and Professional Development

One of the requirements of professional practice is the maintenance of competence. Each practitioner is responsible for devising and implementing professional development strategies. The Academy of Nutrition and Dietetics' Professional Development Committee developed a philosophy statement to assist members in their efforts to develop personal professional development plans.

The rapidly changing character and increasing complexity of dietetics practice demands continual updating of the practitioner's knowledge, skills, and understanding. Professional development recognizes an individual's investment of time and effort required for exemplary professional performance throughout a career. Personal professional development is the lifelong process of active participation in learning activities that assist in maintaining and advancing continuing competence in professional practice. Professional development begins within the entry-level educational program and continues throughout the career of the dietetics professional (**Figure 10–2**).[3]

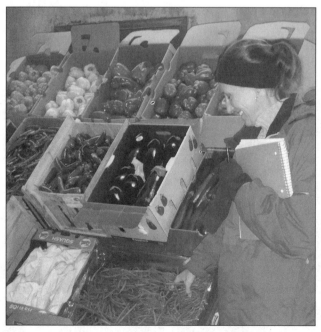

FIGURE 10–2 A student learns how to select fresh produce on a trip to the wholesale market.
Courtesy of Lari Bright

The Academy's strategic plan identifies lifelong learning as one of the values on which the future of dietetics will be built. The role of the CDR and the Professional Development Portfolio in ensuring practitioner competence were discussed in Chapters 4, 5 and 7.

Standards of Professional Practice

The phrase "Standards of Professional Practice,"[4] as used by the Academy, refers to a set of defined statements of a dietetic professional's responsibility for providing services, regardless of the setting, project, case, or situation. There are six standards. Each standard has a rationale statement, a list of indicators that this standard is being met, and examples of outcomes when the standard is met. Thus, the standards provide individual practitioners with a systematic plan for implementing, evaluating, and adjusting performance in any area of practice. The six standards, which are listed on the Academy of Nutrition and Dietetics' website at www.eatright.org, and discussed in Chapter 7 describe the key characteristics of the dietetic profession and focus on the results or outcomes of services.

Professional Ethics

Ethical issues[5] faced by members of the dietetics profession are as diverse as the settings in which members practice. In medical and clinical settings, patients' rights, confidentiality of information, and the provision of food and water are the primary issues that must be confronted. In foodservice settings, ethical issues revolve around the management of money, personnel, materials, and time. In research and education, issues of plagiarism and research designs involving animals or human beings are issues of ethical concern.

Every professional association must address the issue of acceptable professional behavior. This is usually accomplished through a written document called a code of ethics. The code describes the philosophy and expectations of conduct to which the association agrees its members should adhere. The Code of Ethics for the Profession of Dietetics can be found on the Academy of Nutrition and Dietetics' website (www.eatright.org) and is discussed in Chapter 7. The Code of Ethics is voluntary and enforceable. It challenges all members, RDs, and DTRs to uphold ethical principles, and it establishes a fair system to deal with complaints about members and credentialed practitioners from peers and the public.

The purpose of a professional code of ethics is to reflect the principles of the profession and to provide an outline of the obligations of the member of that profession to self, client, society, and the profession. The Code of Ethics for the Profession of Dietetics addresses the provision of professional services, the accurate presentation of credentials and qualifications, standards for avoiding conflict of interest, and accountability for professional competence in practice. The Code also speaks to compliance with laws and regulations concerning the profession; presentation of substantiated information; confidentiality of information; the honesty, integrity, and fairness of the member; and the obligation to uphold the standards of the profession by reporting apparent violations.

New members joining the Academy receive a copy of the Code of Ethics and sign a statement stating that they will abide by it. The review process for violations of this code includes a review of the complaint, an investigation, a hearing, and, finally, a decision and recommendation. The respondent may be acquitted or, if found guilty, censored, temporarily suspended, or expelled from membership.

Commitment to the Profession

Those demonstrating professionalism in dietetic practice have a sense of commitment to the growth of the profession, both as a field of intellectual endeavor and as a society in which people of similar purposes band together. This commitment is best demonstrated by active participation in a professional association. Professional associations rely heavily on the work of volunteers at all levels—local, state, and national. Through this collective energy of many professionals working together, an association becomes dynamic and productive. As Peter Drucker said, "No organization can do better than the people it has."[6]

The benefits of professional association membership are both tangible and intangible. The tangible benefits may include receipt of publications, continuing education opportunities, lobbying on key legislative issues, public relations and marketing efforts, public recognition of professional achievements, student scholarship programs, member loan programs, discounts on rental cars and publications, travel programs, association-sponsored credit cards, group-rate medical and life insurance, and professional liability insurance—to mention a few.

Of even greater importance are the intangible benefits that accrue from professional association involvement. The friendships that develop, the opportunity to hone leadership skills, the sense of creative stimulation, the excitement of being a part of the action, and the opportunity to impact issues and shape policy for the good of the profession are good reasons to volunteer at some level of commitment (**Figure 10–3**).

For students, there are additional advantages of active participation. Students have an opportunity to:

- Develop skills in public speaking, writing, and program planning and organizing.
- Network with dietitians, technicians, and other students.
- Observe professional role models.
- Enhance visibility for scholarships, internships, and future employment.

The biggest drawback of active involvement in a professional association is the time commitment required. Frustrations may also arise when costs exceed the resources available for certain plans or when members disagree. But these are minor considerations when one considers the risk of not being involved.

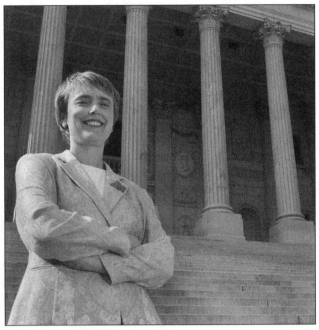

FIGURE 10–3 A dietitian shapes public policy by her advocacy on Capitol Hill.
Courtesy of the Academy of Nutrition and Dietetics

Finally, Some Tips for Career Success

"Whatever the struggle,
Continue to climb,
For it may only be
One more step to your success!"

The Pyramid of Success, shown in **Figure 10–4,** was developed by legendary basketball Coach John Wooden. It took him hundreds of hours of reflection and 14 years of hard work to develop. The boxes on the pyramid comprise the characteristics that Coach Wooden believed essential for success in any and all endeavors. They include:

- *Competitive greatness:* Enjoy the difficult challenges.
- *Poise:* Be at ease in any situation; don't fight yourself.
- *Confidence:* Be prepared and keep things in their proper perspective.
- *Condition:* Mental, moral, and physical condition . . . rest, exercise, and diet must be considered, moderation must be practiced, and dissipation must be eliminated.
- *Skill:* Knowledge of and the ability to properly and quickly execute the fundamentals; be prepared, and cover every little detail.
- *Team spirit:* A genuine consideration for others, an eagerness to sacrifice personal interest of glory for the welfare of all.
- *Self-control:* Keep emotions under control; good judgment and common sense are essential.

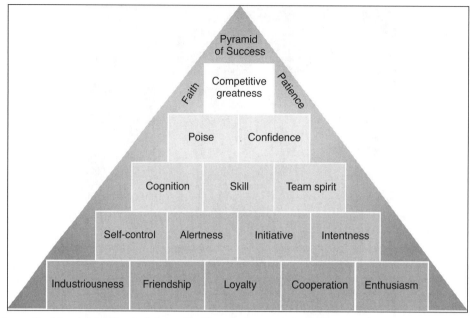

FIGURE 10–4 Coach John Wooden's Pyramid of Success.

Wooden : A lifetime of observations and reflections on and off the court by WOODEN, JOHN R.; JAMISON, STEVE © 1997 Reproduced with permission of MCGRAW-HILL COMPANIES, INC

- *Alertness:* Observe constantly; be eager to learn.
- *Initiative:* Cultivate the ability to make decisions and think alone; do not be afraid of failure but learn from it.
- *Intentness:* Set realistic goals; concentrate by resisting all temptations and being determined and persistent.
- *Industriousness:* Worthwhile results come from hard work and careful planning.
- *Friendship:* Requires mutual esteem, respect and devotion; like marriage it must not be taken for granted but requires a joint effort.
- *Loyalty:* Keep your self-respect.
- *Cooperation:* Listen if you want to be heard; be interested in finding the best way, not in having your own way.
- *Enthusiasm:* Truly enjoy what you are doing.[7]

He also recommends the development of the following 10 qualities for success:

1. Faith, through prayer
2. Patience, good things take time
3. Fight, determined effort
4. Integrity, purity of intention
5. Resourcefulness, proper judgment
6. Reliability, creates respect
7. Adaptability, to any situation
8. Honesty, in thought and action

9. Ambition, for noble goals

10. Sincerity, keeps friends[7]

High self-esteem and open-mindedness are embedded in several areas of the triangle. A positive attitude is a trait that successful practitioners share. Many of these traits are developed, not inborn. As Abraham Lincoln said, "Most of us are about as happy as we make up our minds to be." A positive outlook can be developed in a number of ways. Dr. Wolf Rinke, in his books *Positive Attitude: The Key to Peak Performance* (2003) and *The 6 Success Strategies for Winning at Life, Love, and Business* (1996), offer a number of suggestions including:

- Build a network of positive colleagues—associate with positive people.
- Reformulate your language by using positive words rather than negative.
- When anyone asks, "How are you doing?" answer "GREAT!" with enthusiasm.
- Appreciate yourself for who you are rather than who you think you ought to be.
- Love people for the way they are not for the way you think they ought to be.
- Make it a habit to treat every person you meet as if he or she were the most important person in the world.
- Live in the present—let go of the past.
- Accept that mistakes are part of life, and learn from them.
- In teamwork, do more than is expected of you.
- Spend less time watching television unless it is purposeful and positive programming.
- Spend the newly found time doing something that will enrich you—reading, a new hobby, professional development activities, and so on.
- Use "I" statements, as described in Chapter 3.
- Say good things about people or say nothing at all.
- Smile often [8–10] (**Figure 10–5**).

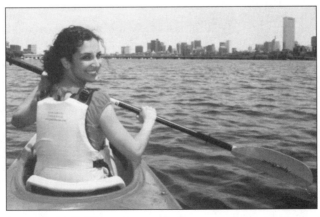

FIGURE 10–5 A dietitian enjoys an afternoon canoeing on the Charles River.
Courtesy of Michele Coelho, RD

Summary

Crossing the bridge from student to professional can be a smooth journey if plans are made early and carefully. Knowing who you are and where you want to go, seeking the advice and mentorship of others, and taking advantage of networking opportunities are some of the ways to make the change less stressful. An internship, graduate school, a practicum, a traineeship, and supervised fieldwork all are helpful ways of bridging the differences between the classroom and the profession.

The profession of dietetics has been shaped and molded by dynamic and dedicated individuals whose careers have made a difference. The profession requires a team approach, with each member of the team being the very embodiment of professionalism—knowledgeable, caring, concerned, respectful, ethical, committed to the profession, and active in the professional organization. The dietetic team member has an essential orientation to the interest of others—the patient, the client, and the community. The dietetic team member is unquestionably ethical in all matters. He or she is committed to preserving the credibility and dignity of the profession and believes that the practice of dietetics has an impact on the quality of life of others. Putting aside personal benefits and/or costs, the dietetic team member recognizes the importance of professional association involvement for the good of the profession as a whole.

Making a smooth transition from school to profession puts you on the road to career success. Know yourself, manage yourself, and motivate yourself—it's really up to you (**Figure 10–6**).

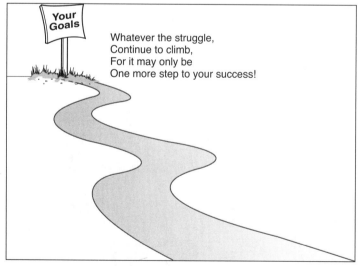

FIGURE 10–6 The road to career success.

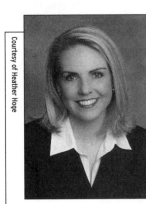

Profile of a Professional

Heather Hoge, RD, LDN

Director of Operations Training
Talent Development
ARAMARK Healthcare
Charlotte, North Carolina

Education:
BS in Nutrition and Dietetics, Idaho State University, Pocatello,
    Idaho
Dietetic Internship, Idaho State University, Pocatello, Idaho

How did you first hear about dietetics and decide to become a Registered Dietitian?
Initially, what attracted me to the field of dietetics was a drive to educate myself on how to eat healthy. Upon taking my first nutrition course, I was fascinated with the science of dietetics and its relationship to the human body. After completion of Nutrition 101, I researched the Didactic Program in Dietetics at Idaho State University. The diversity of clinical practice, foodservice management, community outreach programs, and even sports nutrition made it easy to change from my major at the time, Clinical Engineering.

What was your route to registration?
While completing my Bachelor of Science degree in Nutrition and Dietetics, I took any opportunity to participate and volunteer in field-related experiences. Recognizing the competitiveness of the internship process, I wanted to effectively prepare myself for the application and interview. One of the things I did to broaden my horizons was to be a radio commentator with the Farm Bureau Federation to report local agriculture and commodity impacts for the region. Additionally, I was employed as a foodservice worker at the local hospital, which introduced me to the basic concepts of food production and management. I was delighted to be accepted into the dietetic internship at Idaho State.

What are some examples of your professional involvement?
- Member of the Academy of Nutrition and Dietetics
- Member of ASQ (American Society for Quality)
- Member of ARAMARK's Carolina's Star Team (community involvement)

Briefly describe your career path in dietetics. What are you doing now?
In 1999, I was fortunate to have the opportunity to work as an acute-care clinical dietitian in St. Thomas, U.S. Virgin Islands. While living on the island and working at the local hospital, I noticed that preventive treatment and education routinely began after patients were discharged. Realizing that patients could often avoid hospitalization if they had taken more preventive measures specifically in the area of nutrition, I developed my own consulting firm. This opportunity expanded into providing medical nutrition therapy to four physician offices, two long-term care facilities, and one home healthcare agency.

One of my more exciting endeavors included two radio broadcasts to increase community awareness around nutrition. The first was a 5-minute prerecorded session that provided the local community and surrounding islands with interesting facts and tips about nutrition. The second "Health Matters," which I cohosted, allowed residents to call in and ask nutrition-related questions based on the program topics, such as diabetes, renal disease, and weight control.

After 5 years of living in the Caribbean, I headed to Durham, North Carolina, where I was hired as the Assistant Director of Patient Services at Duke University Hospital. While at Duke, my role switched from a clinical focus to that of foodservice management. After successful implementation of several programs, including a patient menu with advanced diet office technology, a state-of-the-art meal delivery system, and development of performance and quality improvement programs, I was promoted to the role of Director of Food and Nutrition at Durham Regional Hospital.

In 2007, I was promoted to Director of Operations for ARAMARK Healthcare Food Services. In this position, I assumed responsibility for business development, with a focus on managing by metrics, training, compliance assessment, divisional program development, and innovation.

In February 2010, my diverse dietetics career and experiences led me in yet another direction within the organization. As Director of Operations Training, I focus on the development of operational training platforms for ARAMARK Healthcare managers. I am responsible for ensuring our managers fully understand the requirements, characteristics, and attributes necessary to effectively deliver operational excellence and service to achieve our organizational goals.

What excites you about dietetics and the future of our profession?

As you can see from my journey, career opportunities in the field of dietetics are limitless. When I started, I was solely focused on the clinical aspect of nutrition. Never in my wildest imagination did I foresee my career evolving in the direction of training and development. Now is an exciting time to be in the profession of dietetics. Whether it is an active voice in healthcare reform, a sports nutritionist preparing meal plans for high-performance athletes, or a professional resource to your local community, the opportunities are endless. Let your drive, optimism, and imagination lead you on the "road" you want to travel.

Why/how is teamwork important to you in your position? How have you been involved in team projects?

Teamwork is crucial in every aspect of dietetics, from clinical management to foodservice management and beyond. Imagine a wound-healing team without a physician, nurse, dietitian, or social worker! One person alone could not effectively treat the patient. However, as a team, each of these professionals contributes specific treatment suggestions and works in collaboration to improve patient outcomes.

I have been involved in countless team projects, from the implementation of a new food-delivery system at Duke University Hospital to reducing the number of foodservice employee–related injuries within the workplace. I have worked with colleagues on the development of operational training platforms for the organization as well as for our business partners. My current role relies heavily on the thoughts, vision, and creativity of different teams to achieve our organizational goals and outcomes. Teamwork contributes to faster learner, creative participation, innovative solutions, reinforcement for individual ideas, distribution of workload and, ultimately, job satisfaction.

What words of wisdom do you have for future dietetics professionals?

Have an open mind! Be open to focusing on all the aspects of our profession versus one key area. Our opportunities for professional advancement are limitless. Always know your individual resources and don't hesitate to ask questions. It is often not what you know but whom you can contact to obtain the information.

Keep in mind that every individual within an organization is crucial to its success, whether it be the dishwasher in the kitchen or the CEO of an organization; therefore, treat everyone with respect. For example, when I was in the Virgin Islands, I learned that it is considered extremely rude if you do not greet people you come across with "Good morning," "Good afternoon," or "Good evening." Even when entering an office full of strangers, the expectation is to greet all individuals. When I returned to the States, I continued this courtesy in my professional environment and said "Good morning" to every one of my employees. This reception made the employees feel appreciated and provided a means for consistent communication.

Network and build rapport with individuals within your own professional family. Relationships and communication are the keys to success. Don't be afraid to make a mistake. We all do, and often we learn more from those mistakes than we do when everything is going perfectly!

Suggested Activities

1. Begin to research internship opportunities for Dietetic Technician Programs. What characteristics of a program are important to you? Location, graduate credits, opportunity to specialize, number of interns accepted in each class, cost, length of program? Visit the Academy of Nutrition and Dietetics website at www.eatright.org, and click "Become an RD or DTR." then click "Accredited Programs." Choose at least five internship programs or Dietetic Technician Programs and send for their information packets. Compare the programs with your preferences.

2. Want to learn more success strategies? Go to www.wolfrinke.com and click "Make It a Winning Life eNewsletter." Scroll down to the January–February 2012 issue of the newsletter and read through the articles. What strategies would you be willing to incorporate into your life at school and work? What ideas were new to you? How might you adapt them for your own use?

3. More good advice is available at www.rgba.com/article_career_success .htm. Read the short article on career success strategies. What new strategy did you learn about that you might be willing to try?

4. What's the job market like? Go to www.monster.com. Search for the keyword "dietitian" or "dietetic technician"; in the location box, enter your state. How many positions were listed? Choose one of the positions that you might be interested in sometime in the future. Click the position to find out more about it.

5. The ability to network is important throughout a professional career. Visit https:www.career.Berkeley.edu and search "networking tips." Read the short article on the art of networking. At www.mindtools .com, search for "listening" and watch the short video on listening skills. This is a good reminder of the importance of active listening for good communication.

6. Visit your school's library to determine which nutrition periodicals are available. Carefully examine at least one issue of each, and write one or two sentences describing the journal. For example, one publication might be described as a monthly publication with literature reviews of nutrition research and occasional book reviews. Frequently, many articles in an issue are related to the same topic.

7. Carefully examine an issue of a popular magazine that contains articles on nutrition, such as *Shape* or *Prevention*. Briefly evaluate the reliability and validity of the nutrition content.

8. Attend a continuing education program sponsored by a local dietetic association. Write a report describing what is required of attendees to obtain continuing education credit.

9. Discuss the following scenario: A private-practice dietitian regularly recommends that clients take megadoses of several vitamins. The dietitian bases the recommendation on years of research by a scientist who

has testimonial evidence that the treatment works for a number of medical conditions. The dietitian's clients claim to have been helped when traditional medicine has failed. Has the Code of Ethics been violated? What are the issues here?

10. As a follow-up to Activity 9, go to www.eatright/codeofethics.org, click the "Become an RD or DTR" link, scroll to the bottom of the page, and then click "Commission on Dietetic Registration." At the CDR page, click on Products, Services, and Resources. Under the "Resources" heading click the "2009 Code of Ethics." Read at least the first page of this article. Based on this information, would you change the answer that you gave for Activity 9?

Selected Websites

- http://careerplanning.about.com—Career planning resources at About.com.
- www.CoachWooden.com—Pyramid of Success developed by John Wooden.

Suggested Readings

Abraham J. *Getting Everything You Can Out of All You've Got.* New York: St. Martin's Press; 2000.

Biesemeier C, Marino L, Schofield MK, eds. *Connective Leadership.* Chicago: American Dietetic Association; 2000.

Brandon N. *Self-Esteem at Work.* San Francisco: Jossey-Bass; 1998.

Cherniss C. Emotional Intelligence: What It Is and Why It Matters. Consortium for Research on Emotional Intelligence in Organizations website. http://www.eiconsortium.org/reports/what_is_emotional_intelligence.html. Accessed February 19, 2013.

Drucker P. Managing oneself. *Harvard Business Rev.* 1999;77(2):64–74.

Goleman D. Primal leadership: the hidden driver of great performance. *Harvard Business Rev.* 2001;79(11):42–51.

Johns Hopkins Career Center for Students. http://www.jhu.edu/careers. Making Career Decisions. Adjust to Transition. Available at: http://www.northshorelij.com/NSLIJ/Dietetic+Internship+Program+Curriculum. Accessed February 15, 2004.

Maillet JO. Dietetics in 2017: what does the future hold? *J Am Diet Assoc.* 2002;102(10):1404–1407.

McKay DR. Why you need a mentor. About.com website. http://careerplanning.about.com/od/workplacesurvival/a/mentor.htm. Accessed February 19, 2013.

Moore KK. Criteria for acceptance to preprofessional dietetics programs vs. desired qualities of professionals: an analysis. *J Am Diet Assoc.* 1995;95(1):77–81.

Nutrition: Master of public health. University of North Carolina, Gillings School of Public Health website. http://www.sph.unc.edu/nutr/degrees/#MasterMPH. Accessed February 19, 2013.

Parks SC. The fractured ant hill: a new architecture for sustaining the future. *J Am Diet Assoc.* 2002;102:33.

Rasmussen K. Charting a Path from Student to Professional. Info Career Trands website. http://lisjobs.com/career_trends/?p=154. Accessed February 19, 2013.

Seligman M. *Learned Optimism.* New York: Pocket Books; 1998.

Trifari J. From student to professional: making the transition. *The New Social Worker* [serial online] 1999;6(Winter):1.

References

1. Pauline Schatz, EdD, RD. Email message. February 6, 2004. Reprinted by permission of the Estate of Pauline Schatz.

2. Moores S. Six heads are better than one. *ADA Times* 2003;1(Sept/Oct):1–3

3. American Dietetic Association. Professional Development Philosophy Statement. Available at: http://www.eatright.org/Public/Continuing Education/100_13033.cfm. Accessed February 15, 2004.

4. American Dietetic Association. Standards of Professional Practice. Available at: http://www.eatright.org/Public/GovernmentAffairs/98_9468.cfm. Accessed February 15, 2004.

5. American Dietetic Association/Commission on Dietetic Registration. Code of ethics for the profession of dietetics. *J Am Diet Assoc.* 1999;99(1):109–113. Also available at: http://www.eatright.org/Public/Index_8915.cfm. Accessed February 15, 2004.

6. Drucker P. *Managing the Nonprofit Organization.* New York: HarperCollins; 1990.

7. Wooden J. Wooden on leadership. Available at: http://www.CoachWooden.com. Accessed March 15, 2010.

8. Rinke WJ. Positive attitude: The Key to Success in Nutrition and Dietetics. Presentation at the Food and Nutrition Conference and Expo, San Antonio, TX, October 26, 2003.

9. Rinke WJ. *The 6 Success Strategies for Winning at Life, Love and Business.* Deerfield Beach, FL: Health Communications; 1996.

10. Rinke WJ. *Positive Attitude: The Key to Peak Performance.* Clarksville, MD: Wolf Rinke Associates; 2003. Available at: http://www.WolfRinke.com/cecredits.html. Accessed February 15, 2004.

Commonly Used Acronyms in the Dietetics Profession

The Academy	Academy of Nutrition and Dietetics
ACEND	Accreditation Council for Education in Nutrition and Dietetics
ANDF	Academy of Nutrition and Dietetics Foundation
ANDPAC	Academy of Nutrition and Dietetics Political Action Committee
ANFP	Association of Nutrition & Foodservice Professionals
AP4	Approved Pre-Professional Practice Program
APC	Academy Position Committee
ASPA	Association of Specialized and Professional Accreditors
ASPEN	American Society of Parenteral and Enteral Nutrition
BHN	Behavioral Health Nutrition (DPG)
BOD	Board of Directors
CADN	Chinese Americans in Dietetics and Nutrition (MIG)
CCN	Certified Clinical Nutritionist
CDE	Certified Diabetes Educator
CD-HCF	Consultant Dietitians in Health Care Facilities (DPG)
CDM, CFPP	Certified Dietary Manager, Certified Food Protection Professional (these two are always used together)
CDR	Commission on Dietetic Registration
CEO	Chief Executive Officer
CFSP	Certified Foodservice Professional
CHES	Certified Health Education Specialist
CNA	Certified Nursing Assistant
CNM	Clinical Nutritional Management (DPG)
CNS	Certified Nutrition Specialist
CNSC	Certified Nutrition Support Clinician
CNSD	Certified Nutrition Support Dietitian
CORPA	Commission on Recognition of Postsecondary Accreditation
CP	Coordinated Program in Dietetics
CPE	Continuing Professional Education
CPEU	Continuing Professional Education Units
CPI	Council on Profession Issues
CSG	Board Certified Specialist in Gerontological Nutrition
CSO	Board Certified Specialist in Oncology Nutrition
CSP	Board Certified Specialist in Pediatric Nutrition
CSR	Board Certified Specialist in Renal Nutrition
CSSD	Board Certified Specialist in Sports Dietetics
DBC	Dietitians in Business and Communications (DPG)
DC	Doctor of Chiropractic
DCE	Diabetes Care and Education (DPG)
DDPD	Dietetics in Developmental and Psychiatric Disorders (DPG)

DGCP	Dietitians in General Clinical Practice (DPG)
DHCC	Dietetics in Health Care Communities (DPG)
DI	Dietetic Internship
DICAS	Dietetic Internship Centralized Application System
DM	Dietary Manager
DNS	Dietitians in Nutrition Support (DPG)
DO	Doctor of Osteopathy
DPD	Didactic Program in Dietetics
DPG	Dietetic Practice Group
DPM&R	Dietetics in Physical Medicine and Rehabilitation (DPG)
DT	Dietetic Technician
DTP	Dietetic Technicians in Practice (DPG)
DTR	Dietetic Technician, Registered
EAC	Exhibitor Advisory Council
EFNEP	Expanded Food and Nutrition Education Program
EML	Electronic Mailing List
FADA	Fellow of the American Dietetic Association
FADAN	Filipino American Dietitians and Nutritionists (MIG)
FCP	Food and Culinary Professionals (DPG)
FNCE	Food and Nutrition Conference and Exhibition
FPND	Fifty Plus in Nutrition and Dietetics (MIG)
GN	Gerontological Nutritionists (DPG)
GRL	Grassroots Liaison
HA	Health Aging (DPG)
HEC	House Executive Committee
HEN	Hunger and Environmental Nutrition (DPG)
HLT	HOD Leadership Team
HMO	Health Maintenance Organization
HOD	House of Delegates
IDN	Infectious Diseases Nutrition (DPG)
ISPPs	Individualized Supervised Practice Pathways
JAND	*Journal of the Academy of Nutrition and Dietetics*
LD	Licensed Dietitian
LDN	Licensed Dietitian/Nutritionist
LHDN	Latinos and Hispanics in Dietetics and Nutrition (MIG)
LL	Legislative Leader
LNC	Legislative Network Coordinator
LPN	Licensed Practical Nurse
LVN	Licensed Vocational Nurse
MCO	Managed Care Organization
MD	Medical Doctor
MDN	Muslims in Dietetics and Nutrition (MIG)
MFNS	Management in Food and Nutrition Systems (DPG)
MIG	Member Interest Group
MNPG	Medical Nutrition Practice Group (DPG)
MSW	Master's Degree in Social Work
MVC	Member Value Committee
NCC	Nutrition in Complementary Care (DPG)
NCP	Nutrition Care Process
NDEP	Nutrition and Dietetic Educators and Preceptors
NE	Nutrition Entrepreneurs (DPG)
NEHP	Nutrition Educators of Health Professionals (DPG)
NEP	Nutrition Education for the Public (DPG)
NET/NETP	Nutrition Education and Training Program
NNM	National Nutrition Month
NNN	Nationwide Nutrition Network

NOBDN	National Organization of Blacks in Dietetics and Nutrition (MIG)
NOMN	National Organization of Men in Nutrition (MIG)
NSI	Nutrition Screening Initiative
NSPS	Nutrition Services Payment Systems (Reimbursement)
OA	Overeaters Anonymous
ODY	Outstanding Dietitian of the Year
ON DPG	Oncology Nutrition (DPG)
OT	Occupational Therapist/Therapy
PA	Physician Assistant
PHCN	Public Health/Community Nutrition (DPG)
PID	Professional Issues Delegates
PNPG	Pediatric Nutrition (DPG)
POW	Program of Work
PT	Physical Therapist/Therapy
QM	Quality Management
RD	Registered Dietitian
RDPG	Renal Dietitians (DPG)
RDTY	Recognized Dietetic Technician of the Year
RN	Registered Nurse
RNP	Registered Nurse Practitioner
RPG	Research (DPG)
RYDY	Recognized Young Dietitian of the Year
SAC	State Associations Committee
SCAN	Sports, Cardiovascular, and Wellness Nutritionists (DPG)
SDA	Student Dietetic Association
SFNS	School Foodservice and Nutrition Specialist
SGA	State Government Affairs
SNE	Society of Nutrition Education
SNS	School Nutrition Services (DPG)
SOE	Standards of Education
SOPP	Standards of Professional Practice
TOPS	Take Off Pounds Sensibly
TJC	The Joint Commission
USDA	United States Department of Agriculture
USDE	United States Department of Education
VN	Vegetarian Nutrition (DPG)
WIC	Women, Infants, and Children
WH	Women's Health (DPG)
WM	Weight Management (DPG)

Index